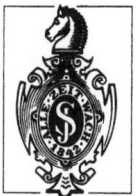

H.-G. Meerpohl   A. Pfleiderer
Ch. Z. Profous (Hrsg.)

Das Ovarialkarzinom

1 Tumorbiologie, Screening, Staging

Mit 65 Abbildungen und 24 Tabellen

AGO
Arbeitsgemeinschaft für
Gynäkologische Onkologie

Springer-Verlag
Berlin Heidelberg New York
London Paris Tokyo
Hong Kong Barcelona
Budapest

PD Dr. med. Hans-Gerhard Meerpohl
Prof. Dr. med. Albrecht Pfleiderer
Universitäts-Frauenklinik
Hugstetter Straße 55, W-7800 Freiburg

Dr. Christian Z. Profous
Farmitalia Carlo Erba GmbH
Merzhauser Straße 112, W-7800 Freiburg

ISBN-13:978-3-540-56405-8

Die Deutsche Bibliothek – CIP-Einheitsaufnahme

Das Ovarialkarzinom / AGO, Arbeitsgemeinschaft für Gynäkologische Onkologie. H.-G. Meerpohl... – Berlin ; Heidelberg ; New York ; London ; Paris ; Tokyo ; Hong Kong ; Barcelona ; Budapest : Springer
NE: Meerpohl, Hans-Gerd [Hrsg.]; Arbeitsgemeinschaft für Gynäkologische Onkologie
1. Tumorbiologie, Screening, staging : mit 24 Tabellen. – 1993
ISBN-13:978-3-540-56405-8   e-ISBN-13:978-3-642-78041-7
DOI: 10.1007/978-3-642-78041-7

Dieses Werk ist urheberrechtlich geschützt. Die dadurch begründeten Rechte, insbesondere die der Übersetzung, des Nachdrucks, des Vortrags, der Entnahme von Abbildungen und Tabellen, der Funksendung, der Mikroverfilmung oder der Vervielfältigung auf anderen Wegen und der Speicherung in Datenverarbeitungsanlagen, bleiben, auch bei nur auszugsweiser Verwertung, vorbehalten. Eine Vervielfältigung dieses Werkes oder von Teilen dieses Werkes ist auch im Einzelfall nur in den Grenzen der gesetzlichen Bestimmungen des Urheberrechtsgesetzes der Bundesrepublik Deutschland vom 9. September 1965 in der jeweils geltenden Fassung zulässig. Sie ist grundsätzlich vergütungspflichtig. Zuwiderhandlungen unterliegen den Strafbestimmungen des Urheberrechtsgesetzes.

© Springer-Verlag Berlin Heidelberg 1993

Die Wiedergabe von Gebrauchsnamen, Handelsnamen, Warenbezeichnungen usw. in diesem Werk berechtigt auch ohne besondere Kennzeichnung nicht zu der Annahme, daß solche Namen im Sinne der Warenzeichen- und Markenschutz-Gesetzgebung als frei zu betrachten wären und daher von jedermann benutzt werden dürften.

Produkthaftung: Für Angaben über Dosierungsanweisungen und Applikationsformen kann vom Verlag keine Gewähr übernommen werden. Derartige Angaben müssen vom jeweiligen Anwender im Einzelfall anhand anderer Literaturstellen auf ihre Richtigkeit überprüft werden.

Satz und Layout: Reiner Göhrick, Manuskript- & Textverarbeitung, 7630 Lahr

21/3145 – 5 4 3 2 1 0 – Gedruckt auf säurefreiem Papier

Vorwort

Neue Vorstellungen zur Pathogenese, zur morphologischen und biologischen Beschreibung, sowie die intensive Suche nach Prognosefaktoren haben in den letzten Jahren zu einem komplexeren Verständnis der verschiedenen malignen Tumoren, die vom Ovar ausgehen, geführt. Mit Hilfe neuer Methoden konnten eine Fülle von Einsichten in zelluläre und subzelluläre Strukturen der Tumorzelle, sowie Erkenntnisse zum Wachstumsverhalten der verschiedenen malignen Ovarialtumoren gewonnen werden. In der Klinik ging mit diesen Entwicklungen eine Verfeinerung des chirurgischen Vorgehens einher. Neben der radikaleren Tumorentfernung rückte die diagnostische Bedeutung der Operation mit einer besseren Beschreibung der Tumorausdehnung in den Mittelpunkt des Interesses. Eine standardisierte Primärdiagnostik ist heute Basis für jede weitergehende Therapieentscheidung. Ein weiterer Schritt in der Verbesserung der Therapie des Ovarialkarzinoms wurde mit der Entwicklung neuer Zytostatika getan. Die Behandlungserfolge gehen heute deutlich über das früher Erreichte hinaus, bleiben jedoch weiterhin hinter den Hoffnungen unserer Patientinnen und den Erwartungen der Öffentlichkeit zurück.

In dieser Situation erschien es uns wichtig, die aktuellen Erkenntnisse aus Labor und Klinik zum Ovarialkarzinom erneut zusammenfassend darzustellen und gemeinsam zu diskutieren. Die AGO hat deshalb im November 1991 weltweit führende Forscher und Kliniker auf diesem Gebiet nach Freiburg zur Präsentation ihrer Ergebnisse eingeladen. Die großzügige Unterstützung der Firmen Amgen, Bristol-Meyers, Smithkline Beecham und Farmitalia ermöglichten es, vom 20.-23. November 1991 zunächst eine CONSENSUS DEVELOPMENT CONFERENCE ON OVARIAN CANCER und anschließend ein Internationales Symposium durchzuführen. Die im Rahmen des Internationalen Symposiums vorgetragenen, ausgearbeiteten Beiträge können jetzt nahezu lückenlos präsentiert werden.

Die vorgelegten zwei Bände zum »Ovarialkarzinom« fügen sich als gewichtiger Schwerpunkt in die Reihe der bisherigen AGO-Veröffentlichungen im Springer-Verlag ein. Der Firma Farmitalia Carlo Erba GmbH danken wir für die großzügige Unterstützung bei der Realisierung dieses Projektes. Die Herausgeber wünschen sich, daß mit dieser aktuellen Übersicht nicht nur alle Frauenärzte, insbesondere die, die sich der Diagnostik und Therapie gynäkologischer Karzinome verschrieben haben, sondern darüberhinaus alle in der Onkologie arbeitenden Ärzte und Schwestern, sowie forschenden Wissenschaftler angesprochen werden können.

Freiburg, im Juli 1992
Prof. Dr. A. Pfleiderer

Inhaltsverzeichnis

Vorwort
Prof. Dr. A. Pfleiderer V

Teil 1:

I. Tumorbiologie und Morphologie

Die Biologie maligner Ovarialtumoren:
Fortschritte und Probleme
T. Bauknecht, Freiburg 3

Ovarian Carcinoma: Tumor- and Molecular Biology
B. Kacinski, New Haven 7

Der Verlust von genetischem Material vom kurzen Arm des
Chromosoms 11: Ein häufiger Befund beim Ovarialkarzinom
M. Kiechle-Schwarz et al, Freiburg 20

Die Bedeutung des Onkogens HER 2 beim Ovarialkarzinom
C. Marth et al, Innsbruck 28

HPV DNA in Endometrial and Ovarian Cancer
H. Ikenberg et al, Freiburg 37

Zur Immunhistologie des Dysgermions
J. Dietl et al, Tübingen 49

Modulation von tumor-assoziierten Antigenen durch
Cholesterylhemisuccinat bei Ovarialkarzinom-Zellen
T. Neßelhut et al, Göttingen.. 53

II. Tumorausbreitung und Prognosefaktoren

Die intra- und retroperitoneale Ausbreitung des Ovarialkarzinoms
H. Pickel, Graz 63

Follow-up unter Chemotherapie: Welche Bedeutung haben
die Tumormarker für die Prognoseeinschätzung?
R. Kreienberg, Mainz 72

Evaluation of the Serum Markers CA 125, 15.3
and CA M29 in Monitoring Ovarian Cancer
M.E.L. van der Burg et al, Rotterdam 79

Rezeptorstatus und Überlebenszeit beim Ovarialkarzinom
M. Krohn et al, Bremen 84

Cellular DNA Content as a New Prognostic Tool in
Patients with Borderline Tumors of the Ovary. A Second Look
C. Tropé, Oslo 90

Die flowzytometrische Bestimmung des nukleären DNA-Gehaltes
bei malignen epithelialen Tumoren der Ovarien
J. Pfisterer et al, Freiburg 111

Steroid Rezeptoren beim Ovarialkarzinom:
Die immunhistochemische Bestimmung birgt neue Perspektiven
F. Kommoss et al, Freiburg 119

Klinische und prognostische Bedeutung tumorassoziierter
Proteasen in der gynäkologischen Onkologie
W. Kuhn et al, München 130

III. Screening, Staging, Imaging

Screening for Ovarian Cancer
S. Campbell et al, London 141

Dignitätsbeurteilung zystischer Ovarialtumoren
mittels Vaginalsonographie
R. Osmers, Göttingen 153

Möglichkeiten und Grenzen der Immunszintigraphie
in der Diagnostik des Ovarialkarzinoms
R.P. Baum et al, Frankfurt 159

Aussagekraft von sonographischen und computertomographischen
Staging Untersuchungen bei Ovarialkarzinomen
A. Vering, Frankfurt 167

Teil 2:

I. Chirurgische Therapie

Primary Surgery for Epithelial Ovarian Cancer
N.F. Hacker, Paddington (Australien) 3

Indikation und Bedeutung der Lymphadenektomie
beim Stadium II und III des Ovarialkarzinoms
R. Winter, Graz 11

Surgical Treatment of Ovarian Cancer at the
Department od Obstetrics and Gynecology University
of Göttingen, Germany
W. Rath et al, Göttingen 18

Fertility in Young Patients after Limited Surgery
with or without Chemotherapy for Ovarian Tumors
N. Colombo et al, Monza 24

Erste Ergebnisse ultraradikaler Operationen beim
Ovarialkarzinom der Stadien III und IV
A. Both et al, Neumarkt 31

Die zytoreduktive Zweitoperation kann das Überleben von
Patientinnen mit partieller Remission nach First Line
Chemotherapie und fortgeschrittenem Ovarialkarzinom verlängern
P. Speiser et al, Wien 35

Rezidivchirurgie bei Ovarialkarzinomen
G. Teufel et al, Freiburg 43

Die radikale Rezidivoperation des Ovarialkarzinoms
F. Jänicke et al, München ... 53

Isolierte thorakale Metastasen - Denkanstöße zu einem neuen
Therapiekonzept beim fortgeschrittenen Ovarialkarzinom
A.H. Tulusan et al, Erlangen ... 62

II. Chemotherapie

Statistische Aspekte der Planung, Durchführung und (Meta-)Analyse
M. Schumacher et al, Freiburg ... 71

Aktueller Stand der Chemotherapie bei
der Behandlung von Ovarialkarzinomen
H.G. Meerpohl, Freiburg ... 86

Die hochdosierte Platintherapie - Ein Fortschritt
in der Behandlung des Ovarialkarzinoms?
P. Sevelda et al, Wien ... 99

Cisplatin Dose-Intensity in Ovarian Cancer
N. Colombo et al, Monza ... 109

Chemotherapy and Hormonal Treatment in Ovarian Cancer:
Experiences of the EORTC Gynecological Cancer Cooperative Group
M.E.L. van der Burg et al, Rotterdam ... 114

Clinical Studies of the Gynecologic Oncology Group
B.U. Sevin, Miami ... 124

Mitoxantron (MXN) - Ein alternatives Zytostatikum in der
first-line-Therapie des fortgeschrittenen Ovarialkarzinoms?
R. Lorenz et al, Erfurt ... 132

Möglichkeiten zur Erhaltung der kompletten Remission
beim zytostatisch behandelten Ovarialkarzinom
W. Krafft et al, Erfurt ... 137

Treosulfan in der Palliativtherapie
fortgeschrittener Ovarialkarzinome
L. Hoffmann et al, Hamburg ... 141

III. Strahlentherpaie

Current Role of Radiation Therapy in the
Therapeutic Strategy of Ovarian Carcinoma
N. Einhorn, Stockholm 151

IV. Experimentelle Therapien

Intraperitoneal Administration of the Biological Agents Tumor
Necrosis Factor, Gamma Interferon, and Interleukin-2
M. Markman, New York 157

Intracavitäre TNF Therapie von Patientinnen mit Ascites oder
Pleuraerguß infolge von progredienten gynäkologischen Malignomen
U. Karck et al, Freiburg 163

Aktivierung des Idiotypen-Netzwerks für Patientinnen
mit fortgeschrittenen Ovarialkarzinomen durch Behandlung
mit dem MAb OC 125
U. Wagner et al, Bonn 171

The Use of Radiolabelled Monoclonal Antibodies
as an Adjuvant Treatment for Ovarian Cancer
V. Hird, London 179

5-Hydroxyindolessigsäure Auscheidung unter Platintherapie:
Die Rolle des Serotonins bei der Chemotherapie-induzierten Emesis
A. du Bois et al, Freiburg 185

V. Supportivtherapie, Lebensqualität, Rehabilitation

Risikofaktoren und Verlauf der Platin-induzierten Emesis
A. du Bois et al, Freiburg 197

Morphininfusionen in der Terminalphase einer Krebserkrankung
L. Hoffmann et al, Hamburg 206

Lebensqualität bei Patientinnen mit Ovarialkarzinom
nach operativer und zytostatischer Behandlung
H. Meden et al, Götttingen 212

Belastungssituation und Rehabilitation
von Patientinnen mit Ovarialkarzinom
R. Schröck et al, Scheidegg 217

Hormonsubstitution bei hormonsensitiven Neoplasien
M. Breckwoldt, Freiburg 228

Autorenverzeichnis

Bauknecht T., PD Dr.
Universitäts-Frauenklinik,
Hugstetterstraße 55,
W-7800 Freiburg

Baum R.P., PD Dr.
Universitäts-Frauenklinik,
Theodor-Stern-Kai 7,
W-6000 Frankfurt

Campbell S., Prof.
Department of Obstetrics and Gynaecology
King's College School of Medicine and Dentistry,
Denmark Hill,
GB-London SE5 8 RX

Dietl J., Dr.
Universitäts-Frauenklinik,
Schleichstraße 4,
W-7400 Tübingen

Ikenberg H., Dr.
Universitäts-Frauenklinik,
Hugstetterstraße 55,
W-7800 Freiburg

Kacinski B., Prof.
Dept. of Therapeutic Radiology,
Yale University School of Medicine,
333 Cedar Street,
USA-New Haven, CT 06510

Kiechle-Schwarz M., Dr.
Universitäts-Frauenklinik,
Hugstetterstraße 55,
W-7800 Freiburg

Kommoss F., Dr.
Universitäts-Frauenklinik,
Hugstetterstraße 55,
W-7800 Freiburg

Kreienberg R., Prof. Dr.
Universitäts-Frauenklinik,
Prittwitzstraße 43
W-7900 Ulm

Krohn M., Dr. med. Dr. phil.
Frauenklinik St. Jürgenstraße,
W-2800 Bremen 1

Kuhn W., Dr.
Universitäts-Frauenklinik,
Ismaninger Straße 22,
W-8000 München 80

Marth C., Dr.
Universitätsklinik für Frauenheilkunde,
A-6020 Innsbruck

Neßelhut T., Dr.
Universitäts-Frauenklinik,
Robert-Koch-Straße 40,
W-3400 Göttingen

Osmers R., PD Dr.
Universitäts-Frauenklinik,
Robert-Koch-Straße 40,
W-3400 Göttingen

Pfisterer J., Dr.
Universitäts-Frauenklinik,
Hugstetterstraße 55,
W-7800 Freiburg

Pickel H., Prof. Dr.
Universitäts-Frauenklinik,
Auenbruggerplatz 14,
A-8036 Graz

Tropé C., Prof.
Department of Gynecologic Oncology,
Norwegian Radium Hospital
Montebello,
N-0313 Oslo 3

van der Burg M.E.L., Prof.
Rotterdam Cancer Institute,
Daniel den Hoed Kliniek
Groenhilledyk 301,
NL-3075 Rotterdam

Vering A., Dr.
Universitäts-Frauenklinik,
Theodor-Stern-Kai 7,
W-6000 Frankfurt/Main

I. Tumorbiologie und Morphologie

Die Biologie maligner Ovarialtumoren: Fortschritte und Probleme

T. Bauknecht

Die heute führende Theorie der Krebsentstehung geht davon aus, daß die Regulation von Genen, die das normale Zellwachstum und die Zelldifferenzierung kontrollieren, durch Mutationen gestört ist. Diese Mutationen kommen hauptsächlich in zwei Gruppen von interagierenden Genen vor: den Onkogenen, die die Zellproliferation und die Tumorbildung unterstützen und den Suppressorgenen, die diese Prozesse inhibieren.

Zunächst wurde die alleinige Aktivierung der Onkogene durch Mutation als ausreichend für die Tumorinduktion angesehen. Durch Fusionsexperimente von nichtmalignen mit malignen Zellen und der daraus resultierende nicht-tumorigene Phänotyp sowie der Nachweis chromosomaler und genetischer Deletionen in Tumoren bewiesen aber, daß Gene in malignen Tumorzellen verloren gehen, die für die normale Zellregulation verantwortlich sind. Diese Gene wurden, da sie häufig eine den Onkogenen entgegengesetzte Funktion haben, Antionkogene oder Suppressorgene genannt.

In der Zwischenzeit wurde eine zunehmende Zahl von Onkogenen und Suppressorgenen sowie deren Funktion analysiert. Onkogene kodieren Genprodukte der mitogenen Signalkette wie Wachstumsfaktoren, Wachstumsfaktorrezeptoren, Signaltransduktoren und Transkriptionsaktivatoren. Es konnte aber auch gezeigt werden, daß Onkogene nicht nur die Zellproliferation, sondern auch die Stromainteraktion, die Zellentgiftung und die Angiogenese kontrollieren. Die Funktion der Suppressorgene konnte bislang nicht eindeutig entschlüsselt werden. Man vermutet, daß diese Gene wachstumshemmende Signale vermitteln und so die Zelldifferenzierung und die Zellkommunikation regulieren. Die Aktivierung der Onkogene (z.B. durch Mutation oder vermehrte Genexpression) und der Verlust der Suppressorgene führte zu der Hypothese, daß diese Genaktivitäten kritische Vorgänge bei der Tumorentstehung sind. Ein zusätzliches Phänomen der Malignität ist die zunehmende genetische Instabilität während der Tumorprogression. Daraus resultiert eine Zunahme der Genmodifikationen und der Gendefekte während der weiteren Tumorentwicklung, wodurch der Tumor seine individuellen Eigenschaften erwirbt. Dies bedeutet, daß die Genanalyse, die während verschiedener Stadien der Tumorentwicklung durchgeführt wird, zu unterschiedlichen Ergebnissen kommen kann.

Die Produkte der Onkogene kontrollieren als Stellglieder mitogener Signalwege die Regulation und die Interaktion dieser Signalketten. Dies bedeutet: in einem Tumor kann die Expression eines Onkogens durch verschiedene Wachstumsfaktorsignale, aber auch durch eine verstärkte Promotoraktivität (z.b. durch Mutation) induziert sein. Als Folge kann die Produktion von weiteren Wachstumsfaktoren stimuliert werden, was mit einer gesteigerten Wachstumsgeschwindigkeit einhergeht. Die Dauer der Genaktivität unterliegt dabei einer transienten Kinetik.

Eine transiente Aktivierung in Form eines verlängerten, verstärkten oder nicht abschaltbaren Signals hat erhebliche Auswirkungen auf die tumorbiologischen Eigenschaften. In Studien wurden die Genstruktur und die Genaktivitäten analysiert, um eine möglichst repräsentative Aussage über die biologische Eigenschaften eines Tumors und seine Prognose zu erhalten. Die Schwierigkeiten solcher Untersuchungen sind die oben dargestellten transienten Genaktivitäten und die genetische Instabilität. Ein Befund, der an einem operativ entfernten Tumorpräparat erhoben wird, entspricht nicht unbedingt dem verbliebenen Tumorrest bzw. dem Tumor nach Chemotherapie oder gar dem Tumorrezidiv. Daraus folgt, daß die Analyse eines einzigen Gens einer Signalkette kaum die gewünschte Information zur Charakterisierung einer individuellen Tumorbiologie geben kann. Erschwerend kommt hinzu, daß aufgrund der Heterogenität eines Tumors Gewebsproben aus verschiedenen Tumorarealen unterschiedliche Genaktivitäten aufweisen können. Um dennoch Informationen über die Genaktivitäten zu bekommen, die die Eigenschaften eines malignen Tumors prägen, ist es notwendig, die Expression der verschiedenen Onkogene entlang eines Signalwegs zu bestimmen, die Korrelation mit weiteren biologisch relevanten Gengruppen und dem klinischen Verlauf zu bestimmen, um daraus einen Bezug der Gene, die die Wachstumsgeschwindigkeit, die Invasion, Detoxifikation und Angiogenese regulieren, zum tumorbiologischen Phänotyp abzuleiten. Durch weiterführende in vitro Versuche kann in der Zellkultur die Tumoreigenschaft und die Genexpressionsregulation untersucht werden. Allerdings unterliegen die Tumorzellen in vitro der Selektion, so daß auch hier eine repräsentative Aussage nur eingeschränkt möglich ist.

Beim Ovarialkarzinom wurden eine Aktivierung verschiedener mitogener Signalketten und Onkogene, aber auch der Verlust von Suppressorgenen gefunden. Folgende Funktionsgruppen scheinen für die tumorbiologischen Eigenschaften des Ovarialkarzinoms relevant zu sein:

1. Wachstumsfaktoren: TGFα und FGF
2. Zytokine: CSF-1, IL-6, TNF
3. Wachstumsfaktorrezeptoren: EGF-R, erb B2, fms und IL-6-Rezeptor
4. Nukleäre Transkriptionsfaktoren: JUN, FOS und MYC.
5. Suppressorgene: P53, RB-1 und TGFβ

Im folgenden soll beispielhaft die Bedeutung des TGFα/EGF-R Signalwegs für das Ovarialkarzinom dargestellt werden. Der Wachstumsfaktor TGFα bindet an den EGF-R und aktiviert über second messenger die im Zellkern gelegenen Transkriptionsfaktoren JUN, FOS und MYC. Diese Transkriptionsfaktoren steuern u.a. die Expression des Angiogenesefaktors VEGF und beeinflussen die Aktivität der Gene, die die Resistenzentwicklung im wesentlichen kontrollieren, nämlich Metallothionein, TMP-Synthetase und Topoisomerase II. Ovarialkarzinome lassen sich aufgrund der Genanalysen der TGFα/EGF-R, JUN, MYC und Metallothionein (MT)-Expression in verschiedene Gruppen einteilen. In der ersten Gruppe findet man lediglich eine geringe Genaktivität aller Parameter (TGFα, EGF-R, MYC, JUN, MT), während eine weitere Gruppe durch eine hohe Aktivität der nukleären Transkriptionsfaktoren (MYC, JUN) gekennzeichnet ist. In dieser Gruppe ist die MT Expression häufig hoch, da MT direkt über JUN reguliert wird. Die zweite Gruppe läßt sich nochmals in Untergruppen, nämlich mit einem hohen oder einem niedrigen TGFα/EGF-R Signal, unterteilen. Zu vermuten ist, daß beim Ovarialkarzinom die nukleären Transkriptionsfaktoren durch mehrere Signale aktiviert werden. Klinisch scheinen sich die verschiedenen Gruppen von Ovarialkarzinomen zu unterscheiden. Ovarialkarzinome mit der niedrigen Aktivität aller Gene der TGFα/EGF-R Signalkette sprachen nicht auf die Chemotherapie an (no change und Tumorprogression), während die meisten Karzinome der zweiten Gruppe in Remission gingen. Der kausale Zusammenhang hierfür ist unklar, vielleicht spielt die unterschiedliche Wachstumsgeschwindigkeit eine Rolle. Ovarialkarzinome entwickeln häufig und schnell Rezidive, die chemotherapieresistent sind. Dafür könnten Gene, die direkt durch Zytostatika, aber auch durch die mitogenen Signale aktiviert werden, von entscheidender Bedeutung sein, wie z.B. Metallothionein, TMP-Synthetase und Topoisomerase II. Eine für die Tumorvitalität wichtige Eigenschaft ist das vom Tumor ausgehende Signal Angiogenese. TGFα und andere Faktoren induzieren beim Ovarialkarzinom die Expression des Angiogenesefaktors VEGF (vascular endothelial growth factor). Die VEGF-Expression korreliert wiederum mit der Vaskularisierung von Ovarialkarzinomen. Weiterführende Untersuchungen werden zeigen, inwieweit kombinierte Analysen dieser Parameter den Phänotyp des Ovarialkarzinoms und damit auch die prognostische Aussage besser charakterisieren.

Beim Ovarialkarzinom lassen sich aber nicht nur Unterschiede des TGFα Signalwegs nachweisen, sondern man findet auch eine unterschiedliche Expression verschiedener Zytokine und deren Rezeptoren. Die Produktion der Zytokine und ihrer Rezeptoren, vor allem der Zytokine M-CSF (CSF-1) und IL-6, erfolgt durch die Tumorzellen, sowie durch die Stroma- und immunkompetenten Zellen. Es ist anzunehmen, daß die Tumorzellen des Ovarialkarzinoms über die Zytokine mit dem Stroma- und dem Immunsystem interagieren. Zusätzlich werden die malignen Zellen des Ovarialkarzinoms durch die Aktion der Zytokine M-CSF und IL-6 in ihrem Wachstum stimuliert. Dadurch erhalten immunkompetente Zellen wie Makrophagen, Lymphozyten u.a. in der Tumor-Wirt Interaktion eine doppelte Funktion: erstens sind sie in das System der immunologischen Tumorabwehr integriert, über die Zytokinexpression können sie aber auch das Wachstum bestimmter Tumoren begünstigen.

Diese Beispiele zeigen die komplexen Interaktionen des Tumors, mit seiner Umgebung (Stroma, Immunsystem). Dies erklärt aber auch, daß die Vielfalt der tumorbiologischen Eigenschaften durch die Analyse eines einzigen Parameters nicht hinreichend erfaßt werden kann.

Die molekularchemischen und morphologischen Techniken erlauben, bei einer hohen Fallzahl nach Gen-Modifikationen und deren klinischer Bedeutung zu suchen. Als Nachteil dieser Techniken werden regulative Vorgänge, wie die der transienten Expression, die für die Biologie eines Tumors entscheidend sein können, kaum erfaßt. Die Analyse dieser dynamischen Vorgänge kann im wesentlichen durch in vitro Tests in der Zellkultur durchgeführt werden, wodurch die biologischen Eigenschaften eines Tumors besser charakterisiert werden. Beim Ovarialkarzinom kann die Regulation von Gengruppen untersucht werden, die die Proliferation, die Angiogenese und die Resistenzentwicklung kontrollieren. Auch kann die Interaktion der Zytokine mit dem Immunsystem analysiert werden.

In weiterführenden Untersuchungen sollte man nicht mehr darauf hoffen, die Eigenschaften eines Tumors mit einem einzelnen Parameter beschreiben zu können. Vielmehr sollte die Entwicklung von in vitro Testsystemen favorisiert werden, wodurch die individuellen Eigenschaften eines Tumors mehr als bisher erfaßt werden, um daraus neue diagnostische Kriterien und therapeutische Strategien zu entwickeln.

Ovarian Carcinoma: Tumor- and Molecular Biology

B. Kacinski

Introduction

During the normal monthly ovulatory cycle, ovarian surface epithelium undergoes a set of changes including destruction, proliferation, and regeneration which is regulated by many (peptide and steroid) hormones and their receptors. The corresponding genes transduce receptor / ligand signals to alter DNA synthesis and gene expression. Point mutation, rearrangement, or deletions of chromosomal DNA sequences which alter the function and / or expression of these genes might sufficiently perturb normal ovarian epithelial cell proliferation and differentiation to produce benign, borderline, and invasively-malignant neoplasms from normal surface epithelium.

At least some of these genes are the normal cellular counterparts of so-called »dominant« oncogenes and / or tumor suppressor genes whose altered expression and / or function have been implicated in the pathogenesis of a wide variety of human malignancies, including ovarian carcinomas.

Oncogenes and Tumor Suppressors

Several »dominant« protooncogenes (sis; erbB1; erbB2; fms; H-, K-, N-ras; raf; etc.) encode growth factors (cytokines), their receptors, intracellular second messengers (kinases, guanine, nucleotide binding proteins) while others (c-myc, fos, jun, etc.) encode nuclear proteins (involved in the regulation of DNA and mRNA synthesis) whose expression is increased by the activation of these signal transduction pathways. Several tumor suppressor or »recessive« oncogenes (Rb-1, p53, DCC, etc.) encode proteins involved in the regulation of gene transcription, cell proliferation, differentiation, and cell-cell interactions. The end result of functional activation (by mutation or *over*expression) of »dominant« oncogenes and / or inactivation (by mutation or *under* expression) of »recessive« oncogenes is the increased proliferation, invasive differentiation, and abnormal interactions with stromal elements (increased *angiogenesis, immune cell infiltration, fibroblast poliferation*) characteristic of neoplastic cells of ovarian carcinomas and other malignancies.

Alterations in oncogene and tumor suppressor gene structure and function can be analyzed by a combination of cytogenetic (karyotyping, chromosome banding), molecular biological (cloning, DNA sequencing, PCR, Southern blotting, Northern blotting), histobiochemical (*in situ* hybridization, immunohistochemistry) and cell culture techniques.

Cytogenetics

Modern cytogenetic techniques (chromosomal banding, in situ hybridization) clearly demonstrate that the karyotypes of ovarian carcinomas are both varied and complex [1-12] and that this complexity progresses *in vivo* [13]. Karyotypes range from hypodiploid to near tetraploid and include minimally deviant near normal karyotypes to totally bizarre karyotypes with many structural aberrations [5].

Several chromosomes and chromosome regions have been consistently implicated in structural aberrations and / or loss of heterozygosity in ovarian carcinomas. These include chromosome 11 [7,8,10,12], both the long (q) and the short arm (p) of chromosome 17 [9,24], 6q [6,8,9,11] chromosome 3 [5,8,10,12], and chromosome 1 [3,5,6,8,11].

Chromosome 9 short-arm aberrations (particularly at bands p13 or p22-23) [11] may be associated with metastatic phenotypes.

None of the above-mentioned structural changes have been clearly linked to abnormalities in expression or function of known oncogenes or tumor suppressor genes. However, the *p53* tumor suppressor gene — which is overexpressed (and probably point-mutated) in a significant fraction of ovarian carcinomas [13] maps to 17p (band 13) while the HER-2 / *NEU* protooncogene (see below) maps to 17q (band 21). A putative Wilm's tumor suppressor gene [14] and the Ha-*RAS*-1 [9,15,16] protooncogene both map to 11p [bands 13-15).

Peptide Hormone Growth Factors

A variety of peptide hormones and their receptors have been implicated in growth regulation of ovarian carcinomas. One recent report demonstrates that a variety of growth factors, including EGF and FGF stimulate the *in vitro* proliferation of ovarian carcinoma cell lines [17-21]. Ovarian carcinoma-derived cells or tumor-derived lines also synthesize many potent cytokines including TGF-β [17], CSF-1 [22,23], IL-6 [34], TNF-α [18], TGF-α [25,26], EGF like factors [27].

In vivo CSF-1 (and possibly IL-6) might adversely modify host-immune antitumor responses by decreasing the high levels of macrophage *MHC class II* antigen expression [28] required for effective presentation of novel tumor antigens to CD4+T-helper cells.

Ascites Fluid Factors

Ascitic fluid from ovarian carcinoma patients does appear to contain many potent cytokines active on malignant epithelial cells including CSF-1 [unpublished ovservation by B. Kacinski], IL-6 [33], TGF β [36], coagulation factors [36] and an imcompletely characterized activity which facilitas introperitoneal growth of certain human ovarian carcinoma cell lines in nude mice [37]. In vivo CSF-1 and IL-6, produced by many ovarian carcinomas and activated macrophages may act as autocrine growth and differentiation factors for malignant epithelial and last immume cells.

Growth Factor Receptor Expression

As suggested by the above studies, ovarian carcinoma cells also express many different growth factor receptors which mediate responses to a wide variety of peptide hormones synthesized by tumor cells themselves or by host stromal and immune cells.

Epidermal Growth Factor Receptor (EGF-R)

Not unexpectedly, normal ovarian surface epithelial cells express EGF-Rs [26,29,30] and respond to EGF and TGFα when cultured *in vitro*. Ovarian carcinomas often also express EGF-Rs with or without the coexpression of an activating ligand such as TGF-α [25,30-32].

In two recently published studies, ovarian carcinoma cell expression of EGF-R correlated with adverse prognosis [30,32]. However, in contrast, another study [31] suggests that EGF-R-positive carcinomas may actually respond somewhat better to combination chemotherapy, a result which may reflect the observation [33] that EGF renders some EGF-R positive ovarian carcinoma cell lines more sensitive to CDDP, an essential component of most modern ovarian carcinoma chemotherapeutic regimens.

The functional implication of EGF-R overexpression or activation are less clear. EGF-R activation by cognate ligand (most likely TGF-α) may result in increased expression of other genes such as *jun* and *fos* which in turn may up-regulate expression of *metallothioneins* which may alter resistance to CDDP and of *VEGF (vascular endothelial growth factor)* which may stimulate tumor neovascularization able in turn to both facilitate tumor growth and metastasis and to potentially increase delivery of blood-borne chemotherapeutic agents to tumor cells [34].

Macrophage Colony-Stimulating Factor (CSF-1), Interleukin 6, and their Receptors

Ovarian carcinoma cell expression of macrophage colony-stimulating factor, interleukin 6 (IL-6) and their receptors (CSF-1R = *FMS*, IL-6R) have been described by several groups of investigators [23,35].

In two studies [32,45], CSF-1 and CSF-1R (fms) expression was clearly localized to malignant epithelial cells and stromal macrophages of high grade, advanced stage neoplasms and low level *fms* transcript expression was observed in several ovarian carcinoma-derived cultured cell lines. The second study suggested that, in addition, metastatic ovarian carcinomas were more likely to co-express both CSF-1 and CSF-1R than less aggressive lesions [35]. Other preliminary studies suggest that the level of CSF-1R expression in epithelial carcinoma cells may be downregulated by a gene mapping to chromosome 11 [36] and increased by glucocorticoids and progestins [37].

Similarly, expression of IL-6 and IL-6R has been demonstrated in ovarian carcinomas and carcinoma-derived cell lines. The existence of a functional mitogenic IL-6 / IL-6R mitogenic loop has been demonstrated by the application of *antisense* techniques for the inhibition of gene expression in several ovarian carcinoma derived cultured cell lines.

As mentioned, CSF-1 and IL-6 are abundantly synthesized by many ovarian carcinoma lines *in vitro*; and, *in vivo*: Patients with CSF-1 or IL-6 producing tumors have markedly elevated circulating (CSF-1) and ascitic fluid (CSF-1, IL-6) levels which rise and fall in parallel with changes in neoplastic disease activity. Such results suggest that determinations of CSF-1 and IL-6 levels in blood and / or ascites might be exploited as »tumor markers« (complementary to CA-125) of ovarian carcinoma disease progression, response to therapy, or recurrence [38].

Autocrine or paracrine activation of CSF-1R by tumor or stromally produced CSF-1 may result in expression by tumor cells of activated macrophage like phenotypes while paracrine stimulation of macrophages (in tumor stroma or ascites) may interfere host immune anti-tumor responses as described above.

HER-2/*NEU* Expression

HER-2/*NEU*, (i.e. c-/ERB-B2) amplification and overexpression has also been observed in ovarian carcinomas and several recent studies, suggest that HER-2/*NEU* antigen overexpression by ovarian carcinomas may correlate with a poorer than average prognosis. [39,40] However, this finding contrasts with other recent reports of no significant prognostic impact [41,42].

Genes Activated by Signal Transduction Pathways and / or Metabolic Stress-Biology and Prognostic Significance

Amplification of DNA sequences for c-*MYC*, a nucleoprotein protooncogene whose level of expression is increased by many different mitogenic stimuli is found in approximately one third of ovarian carcinoma specimens [16,43,44] and can be detected in archival fixed material by the appropriate application of polymerase chain reaction techniques [45]. The functions of c-*MYC* in cellular proliferation and differentiation remain to be fully elucidated; hence, its contributions to the phenotypes of human ovarian carcinoma is still unclear.

Molecular mechanisms of resistance to chemotherapy and ionizing radiation

Tumor cell resistance to chemotherapeutic agents remains a major obstacle to the cure — *and even the effective palliation* — of ovarian carcinoma. However, some progress has been made in the elucidation of the molecular mechanisms of certain types of intrinsic and acquired drug resistance in ovarian (and other) carcinomas.

P-Glycoprotein Mediated Multiple-Drug Resistance

Although a great deal of attention has been paid to the role of the MDR gene in other cancers, the role of P-glycoprotein drug transporter in ovarian carcinoma remains unclear. A recent study suggests that only one in 14 (7%) of primary ovarian cancer samples express MDR protein [45].

Mechanisms of Resistance to CDDP and other Agents

Many previous studies of ovarian carcinoma cell resistance to CDDP have implicated decreased drug accumulation, increased levels of sulfhydryl molecules [46,47], and increases in DNA repair. The latter two mechanisms may also confer cross-resistance to other DNA-damaging agents such as ionizing radiation and some chemical alkylating agents.

CDDP Accumulation

Decreased CDDP accumulation appears to be a major aspect of acquired resistance to CDDP with resistant lines accumulating much less CDDP [47-49] than CDDP-sensitive cell lines.

Sulfhydryl Compounds

Some increases in levels of sulfhydryl compounds such as glutathione [49,50] and metallothioneins which may interact with and detoxify CDDP are observed in ovarian carcinoma cell lines selected for CDDP drug resistance. However, no consistent relationship is observed between extant of CDDPresistance and intracellular levels of metallothioneins or other sulfhydryl compounds [47,49,50].

DNA Synthesis and Repair

Agents which interfere with repair of DNA damage [46] by inhibiting DNA polymerases α and γ [51] or by depleting intracellular glutathione (i.e. BSO [69]) also sensitize cells to CDDP. However, increases in repair of CDDP-induced damage in resistant relative to sensitive lines has been difficult to correlate with levels of cellular resistance to CDDP or other DNA damaging agents [53].

Signal Transduction Pathway Components, other Genes

As has been already mentioned, ovarian carcinoma cell resistance to CDDP, is decreased by ligand activation of the EGF-receptor [33] as well as by agents such as phorbol esters [54] which activate protein kinase C. The mechanisms which underlie these phenomena remain unclear but suggest that some genes whose expression is altered after activation signal transduction pathways are important to CDDP resistant phenotypes. Results presented at this consensus conference suggest that increased expression of *FOS* and *JUN* (either alone or in concert with ovarian carcinoma cell co-expression of TGF-α and EGF-R) also render ovarian carcinomas more responsive to CDDP-based combination chemotherapy, an observation which deserves further study both at the molecular biological and clinical levels [34].

Assays of Ovarian Carcinoma Drug Resistance

Most studies of drug resistance have focused on studies of ovarian carcinoma cell line resistance to single active agents while much less work has been carried out with primary tumor explants. Clonogenic test systems available in 1991 remain unsatisfactory since most rely on the outgrowth in culture of a very small fraction of the tumor cells whose drug resistant phenotypes may not be representative of the majority of the tumor cells in vivo. In an attempt to better characterize overall responses to chemotherapeutic agents of the majority of malignant cells in tumor specimens, assays (such as the ATP- bioluminescence chemosensitivity assay) have been developed [54,55] which permit rapid assessment of tumor explant responses to the multiple agents to be employed in a palliative or curative chemotherapy regimen. The further development and application of such studies in future clinical trials should be encouraged. Also, the practical importance of heterogeneity of tumor cell response to such agents as CDDP and of tumor cell primary and secondary (i.e. »acquired«) drug resistance require further investigation.

Summary

Based on the information summarized above, the following hypotheses on genetic and molecular biological aspects of ovarian carcinoma can be proposed:

1. Studies of genes (protooncogenes, tumor suppressors, growth factors, receptors) involved in development and progression of ovarian carcinomas suggest that activation of dominant oncogenes and the inactivation of tumor suppressors are the *ultimate* causes for the uncontrolled cell proliferation, neovascularization, drug resistance and abnormal tumor-stromal and tumorimmune cell interactions characteristic of ovarian carcinomas.

2. The ability to distinguish different subsets of ovarian carcinomas by their clinical behavior and prognosis (aggressive or slow growth pattern, response to chemotherapy, drug resistance), production of and response to cytokines may allow the development of new diagnostic parameters and therapeutic strategies which block autocrine and paracrine interactions. In particular, agents which interfere with tumor cytokine-induced neovascularization and angiogenesis may have useful (*albeit indirect*) antitumor activities.

3. However, at the time of this conference and the preparation of this consensus document, the above hypotheses require further development and continued studies with larger numbers of cases and (fresh, fixed, and frozen) tumor specimens. The molecular physiology of oncogene and tumor suppressor control of cell growth needs also to be investigated in more detail in ovarian carcinomas, by cell culture techniques.

4. Regulatory and signal transduction pathways worthy of further investigation include:
a.) the TGF-α / EGF-R system with the analysis of TGF-α, EGF-R, c-jun, c-fos, metallothionein, TMP synthetase, VEGF.
b.) the fms / CSF-1 system
c.) IL-6 / IL-6 receptor system
d.) *in vitro* analysis of drug resistance
e.) *in vitro* response of tumor cells to IL-3, CSF-1 and GM-CSF and possibly EPO.

f.) Genetic structure analysis should include PCR studies able detect point mutations and minor insertions, deletions, and rearrangements. Genes worthy of such fine structure studies include are: ras, myc, erb-B2, Rb-1, p53.

g.) Cytogenetic studies in combination with molecular studies concerning the loss of heterozygosity (expecially chromosomes 5 and 11) should be continued and intensified.

h.) Suitable techniques include are molecular biological techniques (Southern, Northern blotting, PCR, RNAase protection) in combination with immunohistochemical and *in situ* hybridization and cell culture techniques.

References

1. Huber H., Knogler W., Karlic H., Akrad M. et al.: Structural chromosomal abnormalities in gynecologic malignancies. Cancer Genet Cytogenet 50: 189-197, 1990
2. Eccles D.M., Cranston G., Steel C.M., Nakamura Y., Leonard R.C.: Allele losses on chromosome 17 in human epithelial ovarian carcinoma. Oncogene 5: 1599-1601, 1990
3. Kopf I., Strid K.G., Islam M.Q., Granberg S. et al.: Heterochromatin variants in 109 ovarian cancer patients and 192 healthy subjects. Hereditas 113: 7-16, 1990
4. Russell S.E., Hickey G.I., Lowry W.S., White P., Atkinson R.J.: Allele loss from chromosome 17 in ovarian cancer. Oncogene 5: 1581-1583, 1990
5. Gallion H.H., Powell D.E., Smith L.W., Morrow J.K. and others: Chromosome abnormalities in human epithelial ovarian malignancies. Gynecol. Oncol. 38: 473-477, 1990
6. Roberts C.G., Tattersall M.H.: Cytogenetic study of solid ovarian tumors. Cancer Genet. Cytogenet. 48: 243-253, 1990
7. Boltz E.M., Harnett P., Leary J., Houghton R. et al.: Demonstration of somatic rearrangements and genomic heterogeneity in human ovarian cancer by DNA fingerprinting. Br. J. Cancer 62: 23-27, 1990
8. Bello M.J., Rey J.A.: Chromosome aberrations in metastatic ovarian cancer: relationship with abnormalities in primary tumors. Int. J. Cancer 45: 50-54, 1990
9. Lee J.H., Kavanagh J.J., Wildrick D.M., Wharton J.T., Blick M.: Frequent loss of heterozygosity on chromosomes 6q, 11, and 17 in human ovarian carcinomas. Cancer Res. 50: 2724-2728, 1990
10. Zheng J.P., Robinson W.R., Ehlen T., Yu M.C., Dubeau L.: Distinction of low grade from high grade ovarian cancer on the basis of loss of heterozygosity on chromosomes 3, 6, 11 and HER2/neu gene expression. Cancer Res. in press, 1991
11. Bello M.J., Moreno S., Rey J.A.: Involvement of 9p in metastatic ovarian adenocarcinomas. Cancer Genet. Cytogenet. 45: 223-229, 1990

12. Ehlen T., Dubeau L.: Loss of heterozygosity on chromosomal segments 3p, 6q and 11p in human ovarian carcinomas. Oncogene 5: 219-223, 1990
13. Berchuck A., Davidoff A.M., Kearns B.J., Clarke-Pearson D.L., Iglehart J.D., Bast R.C., Marks J.R.: Overexpression and mutation of the p53 oncogene in ovarian cancer. Proceedings of the Society of Gynecologic Oncologists: 217, 1991
14. Call K.M., Glaser T., Ito C.Y., Buckler A.J., et al.: Isolation of zinc finger polypeptide gene at chromosome 11 Wilm's tumor region. Cell 60: 509-520, 1990
15. Knyazev P.G., Nikiforova I.F., Serova O.M., Pluzhnikova G.F.: Distribution and rearrangements of alleles of c-Ha-ras-1 protooncogene and their correlation with the development of lung, ovarian and thyroid cancers. Neoplasma 37: 647-655, 1990
16. Serova O.M., Nikiforova I.F., Iurkova L.E., Vinokurov V.L., Kniazev P.G.: Alterations of c-myc and c-Ha-ras-1 oncogenes in human ovarian cancer. Language: Rus.; Eksp. Onkol. 12: 47-49, 1990
17. Berchuck A., Olt G.J., Everitt L., Soisson A.P. et al.: The role of peptide growth factors in epithelial ovarian cancer. Obstet. Gynecol. 75: 255-262, 1990
18. Naylor M.S., Malik S.T., Stamp G.W., Jobling T., Balkwill F.R.: In situ detection of tumour necrosis factor in human ovarian cancer specimens. Eur. J. Cancer 26: 1027-1030, 1990
19. Malik S.T., Griffin D.B., Naylor M.S., Fiers W. et al.: The complex effects of recombinant tumour necrosis factor-alpha (rhTNF-alpha) in human ovarian cancer xenograft models. Prog. Clin. Biol. Res. 349: 393-403, 1990
20. Janz J., Kohler M., Bauknecht T., Wagner E.: Growth control in gynecological tumor cell lines and tumor biopsies: significance of EGF-R state and effect of EGF and TGF-α on colony formation. Cancer J. 10: 323-330, 1989
21. Marth C., Lang T., Koza A., Mayer I., Daxenbichler G.: Transforming growth factor-beta and ovarian carcinoma cells: regulation of proliferation and surface antigen expression. Cancer Lett. 51: 221-225, 1990
22. Kacinski B.M., Chambers S.K., Carter D., Filderman A.E., Stanley E.R.: The macrophage colony stimulating factor CSF-1, an auto- and paracrine tumor cytokine, is also a circulating »tumor marker« in patients with ovarian, endometrial and pulmonary neoplasms. Prog. Leuk. Biol. 10B: 393-400, 1990
23. Kacinski B.M., Carter D., Mittal K., Yee L.D., Scata K.A., Donofrio L., Chambers S.K., Wang K.I., Yang-Feng T., Rohrschneider L.R. et al.: Ovarian adenocarcinomas express fms-complementary transcripts and fms antigen, often with coexpression of CSF-1. Am. J. Pathol. 137: 135-147, 1990
24. Watson J.M., Sensintaffar J.L., Berek J.S., Martinez-Maza O.: Constitutive production of interleukin 6 by ovarian cancer cell lines and by primary ovarian tumor cultures. Cancer Res. 50: 6959-6965, 1990
25. Kommoss F., Wintzer H.O., von Kleist S., Kohler M. et al.: In situ distribution of transforming growth factor alpha in normal human tissues in malignant tumours of the ovary. J. Pathol. 162: 223-230, 1990

26. Bauknecht T., Kommoss F., Birmelin G., von Kleist S., Kohler M., Pfleiderer A.: Expression analysis of EGF-R and TGF-α in human ovarian carcinomas. Anticancer Res. 11: 1523-1528, 1991
27. Bauknecht T., Kiechle M., Bauer G., Siebers J.: Characterization of growth factors in human ovarian carcinomas. Cancer Res. 46: 2614-2618, 1986
28. Willman C.L., Stewart C.C., Miller V., Tao-Lin Y., Tomasi T.B.: Regulation of MHC class II gene expression in macrophages by hematopoietic colony-stimulating factors (CSF). J. Exp. Med. 170: 1559-1567, 1989
29. Rodriguez G.C., Berchuck A., Whitaker R.S., Schlossman D. et al.: Epidermal growth factor receptor expression in normal ovarian epithelium and ovarian cancer. II. Relationship between receptor expression and response to epidermal growth factor. Am. J. Obstet. Gynecol. 164: 745-750, 1991
30. Bauknecht T., Birmelin G., Kommoss F.: Clinical significance of oncogenes and growth factors in ovarian carcinomas. J. Steroid Biochem. Mol. Biol. 37: 855-862, 1990
31. Berchuck A, Rodriguez G.C, Kamel A., Dodge R.K., Soper J.T., Clarke-Pearson D.L., Bast R.C. Jr.: Epidermal growth factor receptor expression in normal ovarian epithelium and ovarian cancer. I. Correlation of receptor expression with prognostic factors in patients with ovarian cancer. Am. J. Obstet. Gynecol. 164: 669-674, 1991
32. Foekens J.A., van Putten W.L., Portengen H., Rodenburg C.J., Reubi J.C., Berns P.M., Henzen-Logmans S.C., van der Burg M.E.L., Alexieva-Figusch J., Klijn J.G.: Prognostic value of pS2 protein and receptors for epidermal growth factor (EGF-R), insulin-like growth factor-1 (IGF-1-R) and somatostatin (SS-R) in patients with breast and ovarian cancer. J. Steroid Biochem. Mol. Biol. 37: 815-821, 1990
33. Christen R.D., Hom D.K., Porter D.C., Andrews P.A., Mac Leod C.L., Hafstrom L., Howell S.B.: Epidermal growth factor regulates the in vitro sensitivity of human ovarian carcinoma cells to cisplatin. J. Clin. Invest. 86: 1632-1640, 1990
34. Bauknecht T., Angel P., Kohler M., Kommoss F., Birmelin G., Pfleiderer A., Wagner E.: Gene structure and expression analysis of EGF-R, TGF-α, Myc, Jun, Metallothionein in human ovarian carcinomas cancer accepted for publication. Oncogene 6: 941-952, 1991
35. Baiocchi G., Kavanagh J.J., Talpaz M., Wharton J.T., Gutterman J.U., Kurzrock R.: Expression of the macrophage colony-stimulating factor and its receptor in gynecologic malignancies. Cancer 67: 990-996, 1991
36. Kacinski B.M., Scata K.A., Carter D., Yee L.D., Sapi E., King B.L., Chambers S.K., Jones M.A., Pirro M.H., Stanley E.R., Rohrschneider L.R.: FMS (CSF-1 receptor) and CSF-1 transcripts and protein are expressed by human breast carcinomas *in vivo* and *in vitro*. Oncogene 6: 941-952, 1991
37. Taylor H., Kacinski B.M., Kohorn E.I., Chambers S.K., Chambers J.T., Carter D., Scata K.A., Schwartz P.E.: A potential role for CSF-1 receptor, EGF-receptor, their ligands, and tyrosine kinases encoded by the *trk* and *neu* oncogenes in human cervical carcinomas. Proceedings of the Society for Gynecologic Investigation, 1990

38. Kacinski B.M., Stanley E.R., Carter D., Chambers J.T., Chambers S.K., Kohorn E.I., Schwartz P.E.: Circulating levels of CSF-1 (M-CSF), a lymphohematopoietic cytokine, may be a useful marker of disease status in patients with malignant ovarian neoplasms. Int. J. Rad. Onc. Biol. Phys. 17: 159-164, 1989
39. Slamon D.J., Godolphin W., Jones L.A., Holt J.A., Wong S.G., Keith D.E., Levin W.J., Stuart S.G., Udove J., Ullrich A., Press M.F.: Studies of the HER2/neu proto-oncogene in human breast and ovarian cancer. Science 244: 707-712, 1988
40. Berchuck A., Kamel A., Whitaker R., Kerns B. et al.: Overexpression of HER-2/NEU is associated with poor survival in advanced epithelial ovarian cancer. Cancer Res. 50: 4087-4091, 1990
41. Haldane J.S., Hird V., Hughes C.M., Gullick W.J.: c-erbB-2 oncogene expression in ovarian cancer. J. Pathol. 162: 231-237, 1990
42. Kacinski B.M., Mayer A.G., King B.L., Chambers S.K.: NEU oncogene protein overexpression in benign, borderline and malignant ovarian neoplasms. Gynecol. Oncol. in press, 1992
43. Baker V.V., Borst M.P., Dixon D., Hatch K.D. et al.: C-myc amplification in ovarian cancer. Gynecol. Oncol. 38: 340-342, 1990
44. Kacinski B.M., Carter D., Kohorn E.I., Mittal K., Bloodgood R.S., Donahue J., Kramer C.A., Fischer D., Edwards R., Chambers S.K., Chambers J.T., Schwartz P.E.: Oncogene expression in vivo by ovarian adenocarcinomas and mixed-mullerian tumors. Yale J. Biol. Med. 62: 379-392, 1989
45. Schreiber G., Dubeau L.: C-myc proto-oncogene amplification detected by polymerase chain reaction in archival human ovarian carcinomas. Am. J. Pathol. 137: 653-658, 1990
46. Rubin S.C., Finstad C.L., Hoskins W.J., Saigo P.E., Provencher D.M., Federici M.G., Hakes T.B., Markman M., Reichman B.S., Lloyd K.O., Lewis J.L. Jr.: Expression of P-glycoprotein in epithelial ovarian cancer: Evaluation as a marker of multidrug resistance. Am. J. Obstet. Gynecol. 163: 69-73, 1990
47. Perez P.R., Hamilton T.C., Ozols R.F.: Resistance to alkylating agents and cis-platin: insights from ovarian carcinoma model systems. Pharmacol. Ther. 48: 19-27, 1990
48. Andrews P.A., Jones J.A., Varki N.M., Howell S.B.: Rapid emergence of acquired CDDP(II) resistance in an *in vivo* model of human ovarian carcinoma. Cancer Commun. 2: 93-100, 1990
49. Mann S.C., Andrew P.A., Howell S.B.: Short term CDDP(II) accumulation in sensitive and resistant human ovarian carcinoma cells. Cancer Chemoth. Pharm. 25: 236-240, 1990
50. Andrews P.A., Murphy M.P., Howell S.B.: Characterization of cis-platin resistant human ovarian carcinoma cells. Eur. J. Cancer 26: 1-23, 1990
51. Schilder R.J., Hall L., Monks A., Handel L.M., Fornace A.J. Jr., Ozols R.F., Fojo A.T., Hamilton T.C.: Metallothionein gene expression and resistance to cisplatin in human ovarian cancer. Int. J. Cancer 45: 416-422, 1990
52. Katz E.J., Andrew P.A., Howell S.B.: The effect of DNA polymerase inhibitors of the cytotoxicity of cisplatin in human ovarian carcinoma cells. Cancer Commun. 2: 159-164, 1990

53. Lai G.M., Ozols R.F., Young R.C., Hamilton T.C.: Effect of glutathione on DNA repair in cisplatin-resistant human ovarian cancer cell lines. J. Natl. Cancer Inst. 81: 535-539, 1989
54. Kashani-Sabet M., Wang W., Scanlon K.J.: Cyclosporin A suppresses cisplatin-induced c-fos gene expression in ovarian carcinoma cells. J. of Biol. Chem. 265: 11285-11288, 1990
55. Isonishi S., Andrews P.A., Howell S.B.: Increased sensitivity to CDDP(II) in a human ovarian carcinoma cells in response to treatment with 12-0-tetradecanoylphorbol-13-acetate. J. Biol. Chem. 5: 3623-3627, 1990
56. Gerhardt R.T., Perras J.P., Sevin B.U., Petru E. et al.: Characterization of *in vitro* chemosensitivity of perioperative human ovarian malignancies by ATP chemosensitivity assay. Am. J. Obstet. Gynecol. 165: 244-255, 1991.
57. Petru E., Sevin B.U., Perras J., Boike G. et al.: Comparative chemosensitivity profiles in four human ovarian carcinoma cell lines measuring ATP bioluminescence. Gynecol. Oncol. 38: 155-160, 1990

Der Verlust von genetischem Material vom kurzen Arm des Chromosoms 11: Ein häufiger Befund beim Ovarialkarzinom

M. Kiechle-Schwarz, L. Walz, A. Pfleiderer

Zusammenfassung

Es gibt zahlreiche Hinweise dafür, daß Gene, die auf dem kurzen Arm von Chromosom 11 lokalisiert sind, bei der Entwicklung von malignen Ovarialtumoren eine wichtige Rolle spielen. Kürzlich veröffentlichte molekularbiologische und auch zytogenetische Untersuchungen haben Deletionen im Bereich 11p beim Ovarialkarzinom nachweisen können. Es ist hinreichend bekannt, daß der Verlust von wachstumsregulierenden Genen, die auch als Tumorsuppressorgene oder rezessive Krebsgene bezeichnet werden, zur Expression eines tumorigenen Phänotyps oder zur Progression eines Tumors führen können. Daher haben wir in dieser Arbeit rekombinante DNA-Techniken angewendet, um die Häufigkeit von Allelverlusten aus dem distalen 11p Bereich bei malignen Ovarialtumoren zu analysieren. Dabei wurde die DNA von 37 Tumoren von insgesamt 30 Patientinnen mit der DNA der entsprechenden normalen Kontrollen (Blutlymphozyten oder Normalgewebe) in der Southern Blot Hybridisierung verglichen. Hierbei wurden vier polymorphe Proben (pEJ6.6, phins310, p20.36, pEM36) aus vier Genen (H-RAS 1 , INS, PTH, CALCA) benutzt. Einen Verlust der konstitutionellen Heterozygotie wurde in 40% der informativen Fälle (12 von 30) gefunden. In neun Fällen konnte zusätzlich ein Rearrangement im h-ras1 Onkogen gefunden werden. Interessanterweise ließ sich ein derartiger 11p Verlust bei den fünf hochdifferenzierten Ovarialkarzinomen nicht nachweisen. Diese Ergebnisse zeigen, daß der 11p Allelverlust beim Ovarialkarzinom ein häufiges und somit wichtiges Ereignis im Rahmen der Tumorentstehung und -entwicklung darstellt. Insbesondere scheint dies eine Eigenschaft der entdifferenzierten Ovarialkarzinome zu sein.

Danksagung: Die Autoren bedanken sich bei den Drs. Weinberg, Bell, Höppener und Mayer für die Bereitstellung der polymorphen Proben. Dieses Forschungsprojekt wird von der Deutschen Forschungsgemeinschaft unterstützt (AZ Ki 352-2).

Einführung

Neuere Untersuchungen haben gezeigt, daß sogenannte Tumorsuppressorgene bei der Entstehung einer Reihe von Tumoren von großer Wichtigkeit sind. Tumorsuppressorgene sind Gene, welche ebenso wie die Onkogene für Proteine kodieren, die das Zellwachstum kontrollieren. Im Gegensatz zu den Onkogenen haben die Genprodukte der Tumorsuppressorgene eher einen hemmenden Effekt auf das Zellwachstum, sodaß eine Zelle vornehmlich dann unkontrolliert zu wachsen beginnt, wenn ein solches Gen nicht exprimiert werden kann. Der am häufigsten beschriebene Mechanismus, der zu einer derartigen Alteration führen kann, ist neben der Punktmutation eine chromosonale Deletion. Somit kommt es zu einem Verlust von DNA-Abschnitten, welche ein oder mehrere Tumorsuppressorgene beinhalten [1].

Es gibt zahlreiche Hinweise dafür, daß auf dem kurzen Arm von Chromosom 11 ein solches Gen lokalisiert ist. Zum einen konnte durch Somazellhybrid- [2] und Monochromosomentransferuntersuchungen [3] eine Unterdrückung des tumorigenen Phänotyps bei z.b. HeLa-Zellen erzielt werden. Zum anderen konnte bei einigen heriditären Tumorerkrankungen, wie beispielsweise Wilms' Tumoren oder Hepatoblastomen, aber auch bei sporadischen Tumoren, wie Blasen- und Mammakarzinomen, solche 11p Deletionen nachgewiesen werden [1].

In dieser Arbeit sollte untersucht werden inwieweit ein mutmaßliches Tumorsuppressorgen, welches auf dem kurzen Arm von Chromosom 11 lokalisiert ist, bei der Ovarialkarzinomentwicklung von Bedeutung ist.

Methoden, Materialien und Ergebnisse

Mit Hilfe rekombinanter DNA-Techniken, sogenannten RFLP (Restriktions-Fragment-Längen-Polymorphismen) wurde die Häufigkeit von Allelverlusten aus dem distalen 11p Bereich bei malignen Ovarialtumoren analysiert. Dabei wurde die DNA von 37 Tumoren von insgesamt 30 Patientinnen mit der DNA der entsprechenden normalen Kontrollen (Blutlymphozyten oder Normalgewebe) in der Southern blot Hybridisierung verglichen. Es kamen hierbei vier polymorphe Proben (pEJ6.6, phins310, p20.36, pEM36) aus vier Genen (H-RAS1, INS, PTH, CALCA) zur Anwendung, die insgesamt sieben Polymorphismen im Bereich 11p15.4-11pter definieren. Für jede Patientin konnte mindestens ein informativer Locus gefunden werden. In 12 von den 30 Fällen (40%) wurde ein Allelverlust gefunden (Tabelle 1).

Tabele 1: Klinische Daten

No./Lab.-No.	FIGO Stage	Origin of tumors	Histology/Grading	Age/yrs
01./028/90	IV	Omentum majus	solid/G3	77
02./071/90	III	Omentum majus	serous/G2	59
03./104/90	III	Omentum majus	serous/G3	67
04./105/90	III	Uterus	Adeno Ca/Met/G2	58
05./134/90	I	Right Ovary	serous/G1	65
06./148/90	I	Right Ovary	endometrioid/G3	60
07./164/90	III	Colon	mucinous/G1	54
08./268/90	III	Omentum majus	serous/G2	78
09./307/90	III	Ovary	serous/G3	75
10./310/90	III	Omentum majus Right Ovary Left Ovary	serous/G2	60
11./500/90	I	Left Ovary	mucinous/G2	74
12./528/90	III	Left Ovary	endometrioid/G2	72
13./550.90	III	Right Ovary	serous/muc./G1	22
14./564/90	I	Left Ovary	endometrioid/G2	73
15./623/90	III	Omentum majus	serous/G3	53
16./625/90	III	Omentum majus	solid/G3	68
17./638/90	III	Omentum majus	serous/G2	44
18./661/90	III	Ovary	Dysgerminoma	19
19./666/90	III	Right Ovary Left Ovary Omentum majus	serous/clear cell/G2	36
20./670/90	III	Right Ovary Omentum majus	serous/G3	43
21./700/90	III	Right Ovary	endometrioid/G2	61
22./706/90	III	Ovary	serous/G1	46
23./851/90	III	Ovary	serous/G1	37
24./931/90	III	Ovary	granulosa/G2	47
25./936/90	III	Omentum majus Ovary	serous/G3	58
26./953/90	II	Ovary	serous/G2	51
27./971/90	III	Omentum majus	serous/G2	69
28./035/91	III	Omentum majus	serous/G3	50
29./057/91	IV	Omentum majus	Adeno Ca/Met	38
30./078/91	III	Right Ovary Left Ovary	serous/G3	44

G1=high, G2=moderate, G3=low differentation; Met=Metastasis

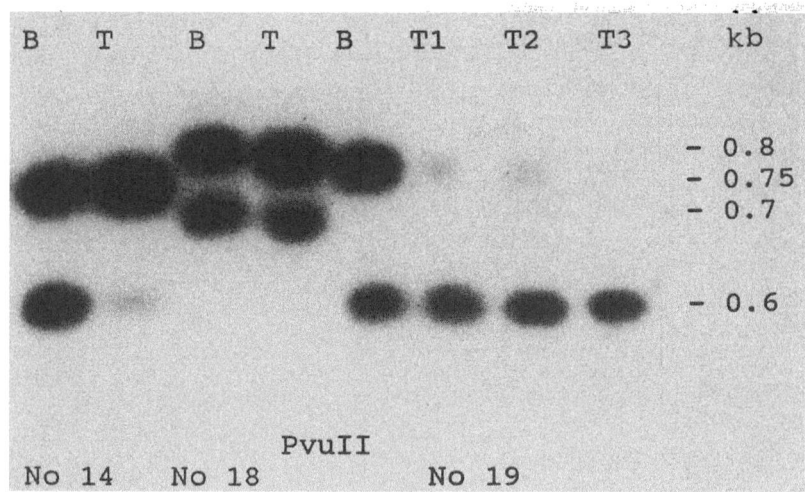

Abb. 1: Beispiele für Allelverluste bei den Fällen Nr. 14 und 19 (B=Blut, T=Tumor, T1-T3=Tumor verschiedenen Ursprungs, T1=Rechter Adnextumor, T2=Linker Adnextumor, T3=Omentum majus)

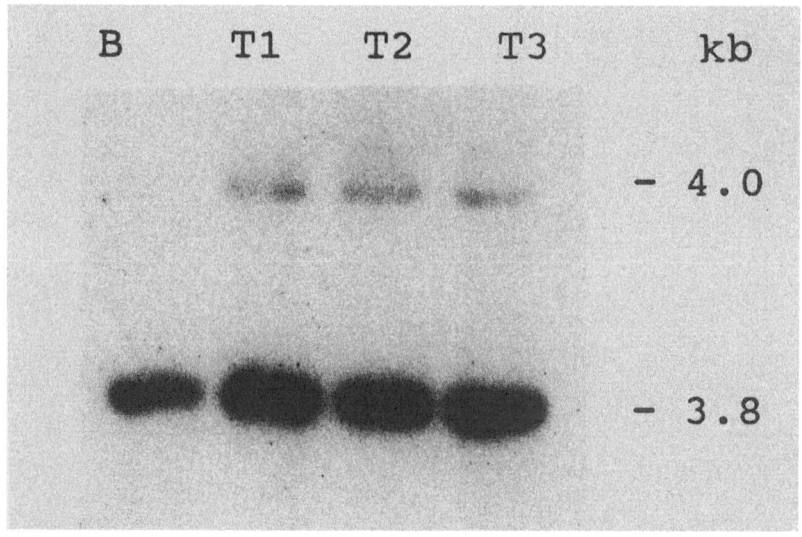

Abb. 2: Beispiel für eine zusätzliche abnorme Bande (4.0 kb) in den Tumoren (T1=Linker Adnextumor, T2=Rechter Adnextumor, T3=Omentum majus) des Falles Nr. 10 bei Hybridisierung mit einer Probe aus dem h-ras1 Onkogen.

Tabelle 2: 11p Allele von 37 malignen Ovarialtumoren (T) und entsprechenden normalen Blutlymphozyten(B) oder Normalgeweben (N).

Locus Probe		H-RAS 1 pEJ6.6			INS phins 310	PTH p20.36		CALCA pEM36
Enzyme		TaqI	MspI	BamHI	PvuII	TaqI	PstI	TaqI
01	B	i	nd	nd	ni	i	i	i
	T	loss	nd	nd	ni	loss	loss	loss
02	B	i	i	ni	i	ni	i	ni
	T	loss	loss	ni	loss	ni	loss	ni
03	B	i	nd	nd	i	ni	i	ni
	T	i	nd	nd	i	ni	i	ni
04	B	i	nd	nd	i	ni	i	ni
	T	i	nd	nd	i*	ni	i	ni
05	B	i	i*	i	i	i	i	i
	T	i	i	i	i	i	i	i
06	B	i	nd	nd	i	ni	i	nd
	N	i	nd	nd	i	ni	i	nd
	T	i	nd	nd	i	ni	i	nd
07	B	i	i*	i	ni	ni	i	i
	T	i	i	i	ni	ni	i	i
08	B	i	i*	ni	i	i	i	ni
	T	i	i	ni	i	i	i	ni
09	B	i	ni	nd	i	nd	i	nd
	T	i	ni	nd	i	nd	i	nd
10	B	i	i*	nd	i	nd	i	nd
	T1	i	i	nd	i	nd	i	nd
	T2	i	loss*	nd	i	nd	i	nd
	T3	i	loss*	nd	i	nd	i	nd
11	B	ni	ni	nd	i	nd	i	nd
	T	ni	ni	nd	i	nd	i	nd
12	B	i	i	nd	i	nd	i	ni
	T	loss	loss*	nd	i	nd	i	ni
13	B	i	i*	ni	ni	i	i	i
	T	i	i	ni	ni	i	i	i
14	B	i	i	nd	i	nd	i	i
	T	loss	loss	nd	loss	nd	i	i
15	B	ni	i	nd	i	nd	i	nd
	T	ni	i	nd	i	nd	i	nd
16	B	ni	i	nd	i	nd	i	nd
	T	ni	loss	nd	i	nd	i	nd

| Locus | H-RAS 1 | | | INS | PTH | | CALCA |
| Probe | pEJ6.6 | | | phins 310 | p20.36 | | pEM36 |
Enzyme	TaqI	MspI	BamHI	PvuII	TaqI	PstI	TaqI
17 B	ni	i	nd	i	nd	nd	nd
T	ni	i	nd	i	nd	nd	nd
18 B	i	i	nd	i	nd	i	ni
T	i	i	nd	i	nd	i	ni
19 B	i	i	nd	i	nd	i	nd
T1	loss	loss	nd	loss	nd	i	nd
T2	loss	loss	nd	loss	nd	i	nd
T3	loss	loss	nd	loss	nd	i	nd
20 B	ni	ni	nd	ni	nd	i	ni
T1	ni	ni	nd	ni	nd	loss	ni
T2	ni	ni	nd	ni	nd	loss	ni
21 B	i	i	nd	i	nd	i	i
T	i	i	nd	i	nd	i	i
22 B	ni	ni	nd	i	nd	i	ni
T	ni	ni*	nd	i	nd	i	ni
23 B	ni	ni	nd	i	nd	i	nd
T	ni	ni	nd	i	nd	i	nd
24 B	ni	ni	nd	i	nd	i	i
T	ni	ni*	nd	i	nd	i	i
25 B	i	i	nd	i	nd	i	ni
T1	loss	loss	nd	loss	nd	loss	ni
T2	loss	loss	nd	loss	nd	loss	ni
26 B	i	i	nd	i	nd	i	ni
T	i	i	nd	i	nd	i	ni
27 B	i	i	nd	i	nd	i	nd
T	i	i	nd	i	nd	i	nd
28 B	i	i	nd	i	nd	i	ni
T	i	i	nd	loss	nd	loss	ni
29 B	ni	ni	nd	i	nd	nd	i
T	ni	ni	nd	i	nd	nd	loss
30 B	ni	ni	nd	i	nd	i	i
T1	ni	ni	nd	loss	nd	loss	loss
T2	ni	ni	nd	loss	nd	loss	loss

Abbreviations: B=Blood, N=normal tissue, T=Tumor, T1-T3=Tumors of different origin (right and left ovary, omentum majus), i=informative, ni=not informative, loss=loss of one allele, nd=not done, *=abnormal bands

Die Abbildung 1 zeigt einige Beispiele der Allelverluste, bzw. Verluste der Heterozygotie. In 9 von 30 Fällen fanden sich zusätzliche Banden, die nicht durch den Polymorphismus definiert sind (Abbildung 2), sodaß man hier ein Rearrangements im h-ras1 Onkogen annehmen kann.

In dem untersuchten Patientenkollektiv fanden sich fünf hochdifferenzierte Ovarialkarzinome (Grading I). Bei keinem dieser Tumoren konnte ein 11p Allelverlust nachgewiesen werden. Darüberhinaus waren unter diesen Fällen fünf Frühstadien (vier FIGO I Fälle und ein FIGO II Fall), die verbleibenden 26 verteilten sich auf die Stadien III und IV. Vier der Frühfälle zeigten ebenfalls keine Deletionen.

Schlußfolgerung

Unsere Untersuchungen haben gezeigt, daß der Verlust von distalem 11p Material ein häufig anzutreffendes Ereignis beim Ovarialkarzinom ist. Der Vergleich mit den klinischen Daten gibt Anlaß zu der Vermutung, daß der Allelverlust bei 11pter-p14 eine Eigenschaft eher fortgeschrittener, wenig differenzierter Tumoren ist. Ähnliche Untersuchungen anderer Arbeitsgruppen an allerdings wesentlich kleineren Kollektiven bestätigen unsere Befunde. Sie fanden einen Allelverlust bei je fünf von zehn fortgeschrittenen Ovarialkarzinomen [4,5]. Darüberhinaus haben Karyotypisierungen ebenfalls eine 11p Deletion als rekurriende Aberration beim Ovarialkarzinom aufdecken können [6, eigene Beobachtungen]. All diese Ergebnisse sprechen dafür, daß bei der Ovarialkarzinomentwicklung ein mutmaßliches Tumorsuppressorgen mitbeteiligt ist, welches auf dem kurzen Arm von Chromosom 11 lokalisiert ist. Ein entsprechendes Kanditatgen aus diesem Bereich konnte bislang noch nicht kloniert werden.

Literatur

1. Stanbridge E.J.: Human tumor suppressor genes. Annu. Rev. Genet. 24: 615-657, 1990
2. Srivatsan E.S., Benedict W.F., Stanbridge E.J.: Implication of chromosome 11 in the suppression of neoplastic expression in human cell hybrids. Cancer Res. 46: 6174-6179, 1986
3. Saxon P.J., Svrivatsan E.S., Stanbridge E.J.: Introduction of human chromosome 11 via microcell transfer controls tumorigenic expression of HeLa cells. EMBO J 5: 3461-3466, 1986

4. Lee J.H., Kavanagh J.J., Wharton G.T., Wildrick D.M., Wharton J.T., Blick M.:. Frequent loss of heterozygosity on chromosomes 6q, 11 and 17 in human ovarian carcinomas. Cancer Res. 50: 2724-2728, 1990
5. Ehlen T., Dubeau L.: Loss of heterozygosity on chromosomal segments 3p, 6q and 11p in human ovarian carcinomas. Oncogene 5: 219-223, 1990
6. Pejovic T., Heim S., Mandahl N., Elmfors B., Furgyik S., Floderus U.M., Helm G., Willen H., Mitelman F.: Consistent occurrence of a 19p+Marker chromosome and loss of 11p material in ovarian seropapillary cystadenocarcinomas. Genes, Chromosomes & Cancer 1: 167-171, 1989

Die Bedeutung des Onkogens HER 2 beim Ovarialkarzinom

Ch. Marth[*], A.G. Zeimet[*], E. Müller-Holzner[*], J. Schatzer[*], M.V. Cronauer[*], A. Ullrich[**], G. Daxenbichler[*]

Einleitung

Die Zellproliferation wird wesentlich durch zwei sich antagonisierende Gengruppen bestimmt. Dies sind zum einen die mit einer Wachstumshemmung einhergehenden Tumorsuppressorgene und zum anderen die mit einer Wachstumsförderung einhergehenden Onkogene. Für das Ovarialkarzinom scheint das Onkogen HER 2 (c-erbB-2, neu) eine wesentliche Rolle zu spielen. Dieses Onkogen codiert für ein Protein mit einem Molekulargewicht von 185 kD, das in der Zellmembran sitzt und alle Charakteristika eines Wachstumsfaktorrezeptors besitzt. Das HER 2 Protein ist charakterisiert durch eine Extrazellulärdomäne, die wahrscheinlich einen bisher noch unbekannten Liganden binden kann, einer Transmembranregion sowie einer intrazellulären Domäne, die Tyrosinkinaseaktivität aufweist [1]. Sowohl in der Aminosäurensequenz als auch in der dreidimensionalen Struktur weist das HER 2 Protein große Homologie mit dem Rezeptor für den epidermalen Wachstumsfaktor auf. Daher dürfte das Onkogen HER 2 auch in der autokrinen Wachstumsregulation eine wichtige Rolle spielen. Somit wird dieses Onkogen auch als prognostischer Faktor interessant. Ovarialkarzinome, die HER-2 überexprimieren sollten auf das Signal des Liganden stärker reagieren können und rascher proliferieren, und dies würde auch eine höhere Malignität implizieren. Die Arbeitsgruppe um D. Slamon konnte kürzlich diese Hypothese auch bestätigen [2]. Frauen mit einer Überexpression des Onkogens HER 2 (immunhistochemisch mehr als 2 ++ positiv) verstarben alle innerhalb von 2 Jahren, während bei Patientinnen mit einer normalen HER 2-Expression die mittlere Überlebenserwartung 5 Jahre betrug. Das Überleben der Patientinnen wurde nicht nur durch die Proteinexpression sondern auch durch die Genamplifikation beeinflußt. So betrug das mittlere Überleben 1879, 939 oder 243 Tage je nachdem ob der Tumor eine, 2

---

[*] Universitätsklinik für Frauenheilkunde Innsbruck
[**] Max Planck Institut für Biochemie Martinsried

bis 5 oder mehr als 5 Kopien des Gens aufwies. In ähnlicher Weise konnte auch die Arbeitsgruppe um Berchuck einen Zusammenhang zwischen Prognose von Ovarialkarzinompatientinnen und Expression des Onkogens HER 2 aufzeigen [3].

Sowohl um die Tumorbiologie zu verstehen als auch um eine adäquate Therapie durchführen zu können, benötigen wir akkurate Parameter für die Prädiktion der Prognose. Die Überexpression des Onkogens HER 2 scheint somit neben den klassischen Parametern, wie FIGO Stadium, Tumorrest, Malignitätsgrad oder Neopterinausscheidung, Bedeutung zu erlangen [Übersicht bei 4]. Das Ziel unserer Untersuchung war es, die prognostische Relevanz des Onkogens HER 2 auch in unseren Patientinnen zu überprüfen sowie die funktionelle Bedeutung des Gens zu untersuchen.

Material und Methoden

Von 38 in Paraffin eingebetteten Tumorproben wurden Schnitte angefertigt und mittels des Antikörpers 21N, der ein Epitop im Bereich der intrazellulären Domäne erkennt, nach Standardmethoden die Immunhistochemie durchgeführt. Der Prozentsatz positiver Zellen und die Färbeintensität wurde von zwei unabhängigen Begutachtern beurteilt. Um dem Problem begegnen zu können, daß bei fixiertem Gewebe Veränderungen des Epitops die Zuverlässigkeit der Ergebnisse mindern, wurden in einer weiteren Serie gefrorene Tumorproben homogenisiert und mittels eines käuflichen Elisa (NEN-Dupont) die zelluläre HER 2-Konzentration bestimmt. Als Kontrollgruppe wurden neben den 33 Ovarialkarzinomen 5 normale Ovarien und 4 benigne Ovarialtumoren untersucht. Die Ovarialkarzinomzellen HTB-77 und die Mammakarzinomzellen SKBR-3 wurden unter den üblichen Bedingungen gezüchtet [5]. Der monoklonale Antikörper 4D5, der die extrazelluläre Domäne des HER 2-Proteins erkennt und dadurch den Liganden verdrängen soll, wurde auf seine antiproliferative Aktivität mittels eines Soft-Agar-Clonogenic-Assay geprüft. Die Beeinflussung der HER 2-Expression durch Interferon-gamma wurde in einem Monolayer-System geprüft und die HER 2-Konzentration mittels des ELISA gemessen.

Die erhobenen Daten wurden mittels des BMDP Statistic Software-Pakets analysiert, wobei nicht parametrische Verfahren (Wilcoxon Test) der Vorzug gegeben wurde. Die Überlebensanalysen wurden mittels des Verfahrens nach Mantel ausgewertet.

Ergebnisse und Diskussion

Bei 16 von 38 Ovarialkarzinompatientinnen konnte im Paraffinschnitt des Primärtumors immunhistochemisch eine verstärkte Expression des Onkogens HER 2 nachgewiesen werden. Der Vergleich der Überlebenskurven ergab jedoch keinen statistisch signifikanten Unterschied zwischen diesen beiden Patientengruppen (Abb. 1). Um dem Problem begegnen zu können, daß bei fixierten Geweben Veränderungen des Epitops zu einer Verfälschung der Ergebnisse führen, wurden in Folge gefrorene Tumorproben einer neuen Patientenserie homogenisiert und die HER 2-Konzentrationen mittels eines ELISA bestimmt. Bei 33 Tumorproben fanden wir eine mediane Konzentration von 2.200 ± 704 HNU/mg Protein, während bei unauffälligen Ovarien (n=5) 785 ± 355 HNU/mg Protein gemessen wurden ($p<0,01$). Auch bei 4 benignen Tumoren der Ovarien wurde mit einem medianen Wert von 820 ± 281 HNU/mg Protein ein gegenüber den Karzinomen deutlich geringerer Wert gemessen ($p<0,05$). Nach Erstellung von Normwertgrenzen durch Einbinden der gutartigen und normalen Ovarien muß ein oberer Grenzwert mit etwa 2.000 HNU/mg Protein angesetzt werden. Damit liegen etwa 50% der Karzinome innerhalb des Normwertbereichs. Auch bei den Patientinnen wo das HER-2 Protein mittels ELISA bestimmt wurde, konnten wir keinen Einfuß der HER 2-Expression auf die Prognose beobachten (Abb. 2). Möglicherweise spielt dabei die geringe Fallzahl eine wesentliche Rolle. Trotzdem konnten wir im gleichen Kollektiv für etablierte Parameter der Prognose, wie Stadium, Resttumor und Neopterin, signifikante Unterschiede beobachten. Interessant war die Beobachtung, daß muzinöse Karzinome mit 1455 HNU/mg Protein einen signifikant niedrigeren Wert gegenüber den anderen histologischen Typen aufwies (2.627 HNU/mg Protein, $p<0,05$). Wir konnten keinen Zusammenhang zwischen HER 2-Expression, dem FIGO Stadium, dem Malignitätsgrad und dem verbliebenen Resttumor sowie der Anwesenheit von Ascites bei der Primäroperation beobachten. Die erhobenen HER 2-Proteinwerte wiesen auch keine signifikante Korrelation mit dem Tumormarker CA 125 und dem prognostischen Faktor Neopterin auf.

Damit können wir insgesamt die prognostische Bedeutung des Onkogens HER 2 nicht bestätigen. Eine mögliche Ursache könnte in der geringen Anzahl der Patientinnen liegen, obwohl wir für das Stadium, den Resttumor und die Neopterinausscheidung auch bei diesen Patientinnen einen signifikanten Zusammenhang mit der Prognose finden konnten. Damit dürfte der HER 2-Expression nicht jene überragende Rolle zukommen, die aufgrund der anfänglichen Untersuchungen vermutet worden war.

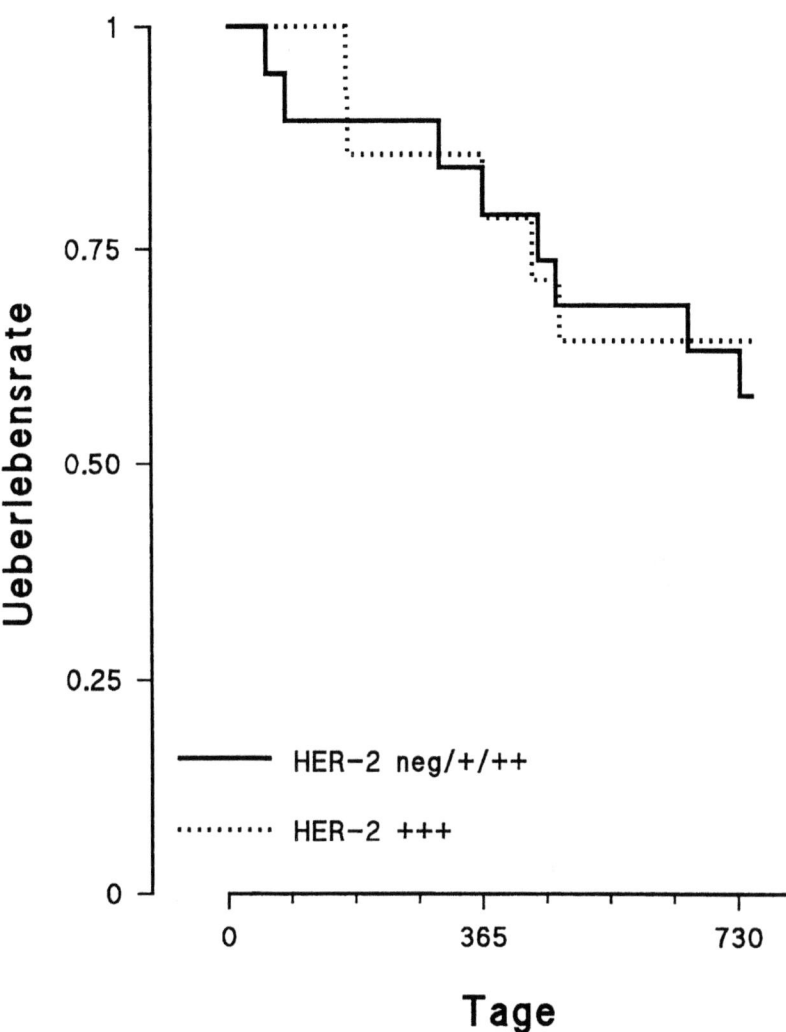

Abb. 1: Überlebensraten von Ovarialkarzinompatientinnen mit normaler HER 2-Expression (1) sowie HER 2-Überexpression (2). Die Protoonkogenexpression wurde immunhistochemisch mit dem Antikörper 21M am Paraffinschnitt ermittelt.

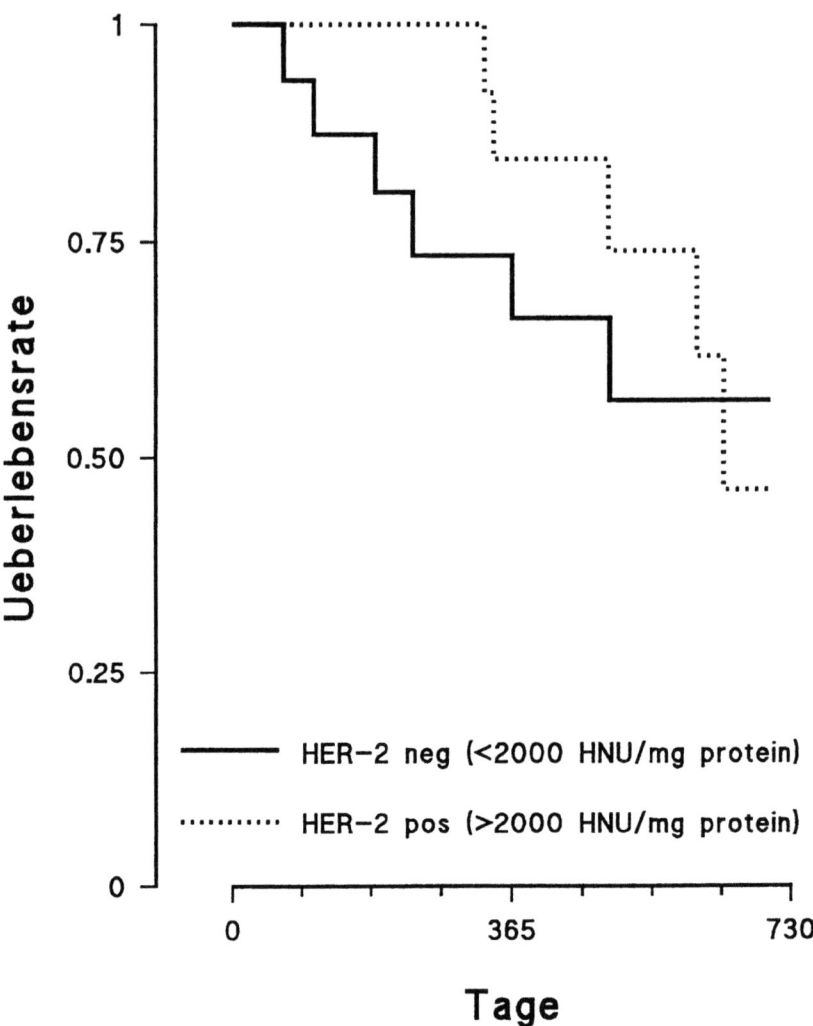

Abb. 2: Überlebenskurven von Ovarialkarzinompatientinnen in Abhängigkeit von der zellulären Konzentration an HER 2. Die HER 2-Konzentration wurde mittels ELISA bestimmt und der Grenzwert mit 2000 HNU/mg Protein festgelegt.

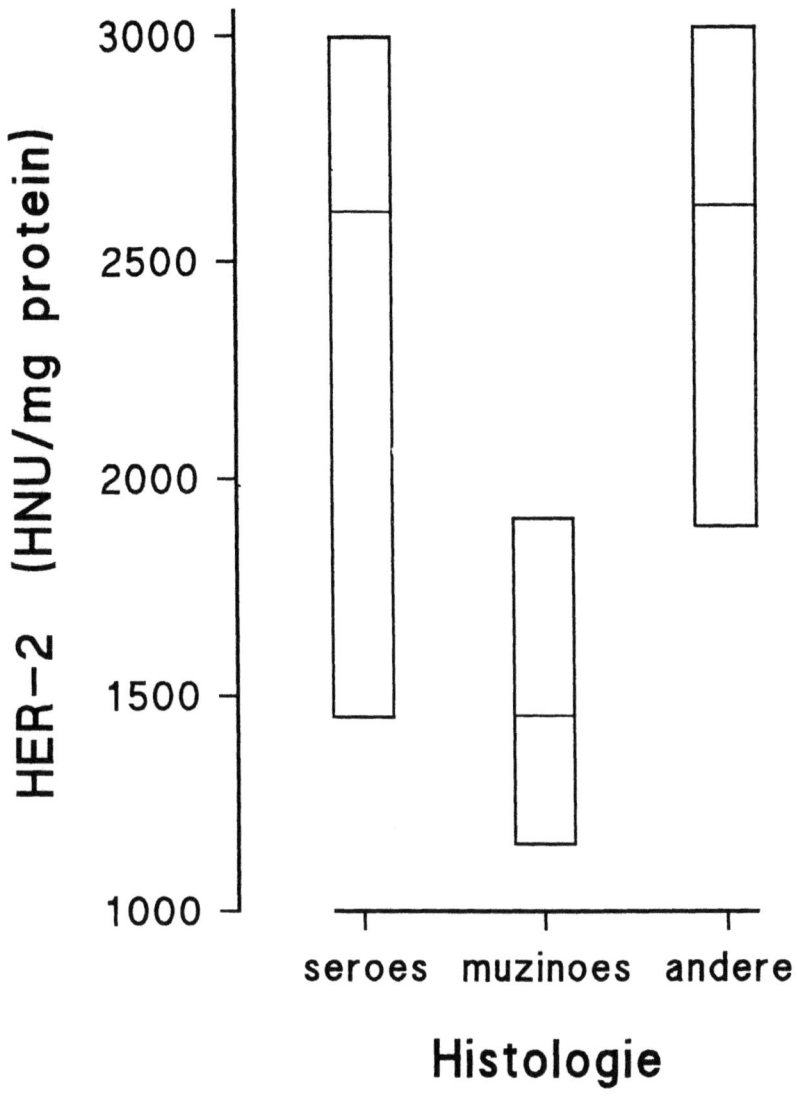

Abb. 3: HER 2-Konzentration in Abhängigkeit vom histologischen Typ. Die Balken entsprechen der 1. sowie 3. Quartile, der Querstrich beschreibt den Medianwert.

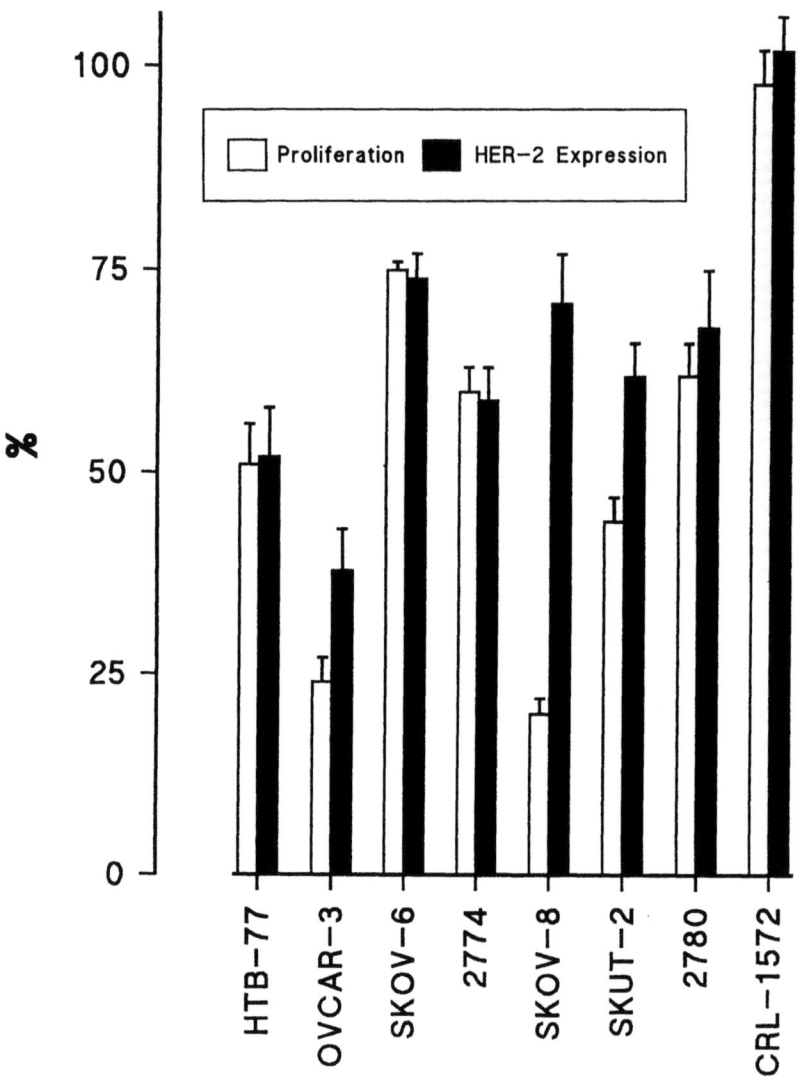

Abb. 4: Beeinflussung der Proliferation und HER-2 Expression durch Interferon-gamma (1 ng/ml). Die Ovarialkarzinomzellen wurden für 3 Tage mit und ohne Interferonzusatz gezüchtet und anschließend die Zellzahl und die HER-2 Konzentration mittels ELISA bestimmt. Die Ergebnisse wurden in % der unbehandelten Kontrollgruppe angegeben. Jeder Balken stellt den Mittelwert mit einer Standardabweichung errechnet aus 6 Proben dar.

Eine weitere wichtige Frage ist die funktionelle Bedeutung dieses Onkogens. Es wird angenommen, daß das HER 2-Protein einen Wachstumsfaktorrezeptor darstellt, dessen Liganden wir nicht kennen. Wir haben jedoch Antikörper zur Verfügung, die an die extrazelluläre Domäne binden und auf diese Weise den Liganden an der Rezeptorbindung hindern sollten. Die Inkubation von SKBR 3 und HTB 77 Zellen mit dem monoklonalen Antikörper 4D5 führte zu einer drastischen Hemmung der Proliferation in diesen beiden Tumortypen (Abb. 3). Zudem konnten wir bei 7 von 8 Ovarialkarzinomzellinien eine Wachstumshemmung durch Behandlung mit Interferon-gamma erzielen (Abb. 4). Diese ging stets mit einer Reduktion der HER 2-Expression einher. Unsere früher geäußerte Vermutung, daß die interferoninduzierte Wachstumshemmung höchstwahrscheinlich durch die Reduktion der Wachstumsfaktorrezeptorkonzentration vermittelt wird konnte durch diese Experimente untermauert werden [6].

Die Expression des Protoonkogens HER 2 ist für die Regulation der Tumorzellproliferation von großer Bedeutung. Substanzen wie die Interferone, die die Expression des Onkogens reduzieren, führen auch zu einer Hemmung der Proliferation. Antikörper, welche die Bindung des Liganden am Rezeptor verhindern, lösen ebenfalls eine Wachstumshemmung aus. Trotz dieser großen funktionellen Bedeutsamkeit stellt die Überexpression dieses Protoonkogens keinen dominierenden prognostischen Faktor dar und wird, wie wir bei einer kleinen Fallzahl zeigen konnten, von den klassischen Parametern, wie Stadium, Resttumor, Neopterinausschüttung übertroffen. Weitere Untersuchungen an größeren Fallzahlen sollten jedoch diese Frage noch eingehender beleuchten.

Literatur

1. Bargmann C.I., Hung M.C., Weinberg R.A.: The new oncogene encotes an epidermal growth factor related protein. Nature 319: 226-230, 1986
2. Slamon D.J., Godolphin W., Jones L.A., Holt J.A., Wong S.G., Keith D.E., Levin W.J., Stuart S.G., Utove J., Ullrich A., Press M.V.: Studies of the HER 2-new protooncogene in human breast and ovarian cancer. Science 244: 707-712, 1989
3. Berchuck A., Kamel A., Whitaker R., Kerns B., Olt G., Kinney R., Soper J.T., Dodge R., Clarke-Pearson D.L., Marks P., Mc Kenzie S., Yin S., Bast R.C. Jr.: Overexpression of HER-2/neu is associated with poor survival in advanced epithelial ovarian cancer. Cancer Res. 50: 4087-4091, 1990
4. Friedlander M.L., Denbo A.J.: Prognostic factors in ovarian cancer. Seminars in Oncology 18: 205-212, 1991

5. Marth C., Fuith L.C., Böck G., Daxenbichler G., Dapunt O.: Modulation of ovarian carcinoma tumormarker CA 125 by Gamma-interferon. Cancer Res. 49: 6538-6543, 1989
6. Marth C., Müller-Holzner E., Greiter E., Gronauer M.V., Zeimet A.G., Doppler W., Eibl B., Hynes N.E., Daxenbichler G.: Gamma-interferon produce expression of the protooncogene c-erbB-2 in human ovarian carcinoma cells. Cancer Res. 50: 7037-7041, 1990

HPV DNA in Endometrial and Ovarian Cancer

H. Ikenberg, B. Schmitt, U. Teufel, F. Kommoss, J. Pfisterer, A. Pfleiderer

Introduction

In industrialized countries carcinoma of the endometrium has become the most prevalent neoplasm of the female genital tract. Most endometrial carcinomas are adenocarcinomas. Clinical experience suggests a division into two main prognostic groups: so called »low risk« carcinomas, highly differentiated, estrogen- and progesterone-receptor-positive and diploid, which are found in corpulent women or after estrogen intake; and less differentiated, hormone-receptor-negative and mostly aneuploid tumors with a poor prognosis [20]. The mechanisms of pathogenesis remain under discussion. Continous estrogen stimulation without compensative gestagen activity has been intensively discussed as a predisposing condition for endometrial carcinoma. Endometrial hyperplasias and well differentiated adenocarcinomas have frequently been observed after such stimulation [25, review see 8]. But the precise role of estrogen in endometrial carcinogenesis is far from being cleared.

In marked contrast to cervical carcinoma, numerous epidemiological studies showed no evidence for any role of a transmissible agent in the etiology of endometrial cancer [review see 18]. This has already been reflected by Rigoni-Stern [21] in 1842 who found uterine cancer (in those days nearly identical with cervical carcinoma) practically absent in nuns. There is an expanding body of evidence linking human papillomaviruses (HPV) to cervical carcinogenesis. The majority of premalignant and up to 90% of malignant cervical lesions contain HPV DNA [review see10]. Anogenital HPVs can be divided into two groups based on their clinical associations. The »low risk« HPVs with the prototypes HPV-6 and HPV-11 are mainly found in benign anogenital warts and low grade dysplasia [29,30]. HPV-16 and HPV-18, the predominant representatives of the »high risk« group are associated with lesions at high risk for progression and with invasive cancer [2,3]. The importance of cofactors in cervical carcinogenesis is illuminated by the high prevalence of HPV-16-DNA also at the clinically normal cervix [5]. A possible etiologic role of »high risk« HPV is underlined by the ability of cloned viral DNA of these but not of the »low risk« HPVs to transform cells in culture [15].

HPV-16 is by far the most prevalent type detected in squamous cell carcinomas of the cervix [3, review see 10]. More than 50% of cervical adenocarcinomas also contain HPV sequences. Here in contrast to squamous lesions HPV-18 is the prevailing type [26,27, review see 10]. The association of HPV with cervical adenocarcinoma is strengthened by the detection of HPV DNA in the majority of preinvasive glandular lesions of the cervix [6,16,28].

These findings and the close anatomic and histologic relations of the endometrial mucosa with the endocervical epithelium make the endometrium a possible target for the HPV infection. Only few studies have analyzed the prevalence of HPV DNA in normal and malignant endometrium.

Ovarian carcinoma is more frequent in women with a low number of pregnancies and no use of oral contraceptives. No further definite risk factors are known [19, review see 17]. Up to now no association between ovarian neoplasia and HPV was demonstrated.

We analyzed 77 cases of endometrial and 18 cases of ovarian cancer for the presence of HPV by Southern blot hybridization and the polymerase chain reaction (PCR).

Material and Methodes

Tissue Specimens
Endometrial and ovarian tissue specimens were obtained at random from 72 patients undergoing surgical and 5 patients receiving radiation treatment at the Universitäts-Frauenklinik Freiburg. In the surgically treated patients, endometrial tissue was excised as far away from the isthmus as possible to avoid contamination by possibly HPV-containing cervical cells. Macroscopically and histologically tumorfree myometrial tissue was taken as internal control. Ovarian cancer tissue specimens were obtained from 18 surgically treated patients. All tissues were snap frozen in liquid nitrogen and kept at -70°C until analysis. Routine histologic examination of the cases was done. The staging of the endometrial cancers was determined by the results of the histologic examination according to the new FIGO classification.

Southern Blot Hybridization
The procedures for extraction of DNA, Southern transfer and hybridization have been described previously [3]. In short, total cellular DNA was phenol-extracted. Two to ten micrograms of tissue DNA was cleaved with the restric-

tion enzyme Bam HI, separated in a 1% agarose gel, and transferred to a nitrocellulose or nylon filter. Hybridization was performed with ^{32}P-random-labelled probes [7] of HPV-11, -16, -18, and — in part — HPV-31, and -35. First a hybridization with HPV-16 under nonstringent conditions (TM -35°C) was carried out to identify only weakly cross-hybridizing HPV sequences distantly related to the probe used. After a wash at stringent conditions (TM -20°C), at which only hybrids with homologous sequences remain stable and a reexposition, the filters were tested at stringent conditions with HPVs -11, -18, and — in part — -31, and -35 sequentially. The probe DNA was cloned in pBR 322 and was separated from the vector before use. Human placental DNA served as negative control. Cloned HPV-DNA was used as the positive control. The sensitivity of detection was estimated to be 0,2 copies of HPV-DNA per cellular genome.

PCR Amplification
The polymerase chain reaction was used to amplify HPV-sequences possibly contained in the tissue samples. Synthetic oligonucleotide primers (table 1) targeting sequences in the L1 region of HPV-11 and the E6 region of HPV-16 and HPV-18 were used. The primers amplified 360-, 120- or 160-base-pair-fragments of HPV-11, -16 or -18, respectively. The type specificity of the amplified sequence was confirmed by hybridization of random ^{32}p-labelled cloned HPV-11, -16 or -18-DNA. The primers were synthesized on a Pharmacia LKB gene assembler by the methoxyphosphoramidite method. The amplification was performed in a 100µl-reaction-mixture, which contained 50ng of cellular DNA, 50mM KCl, 10mM Tris HCl (pH 8,3), 15mM $MgCl_2$, 200µM of each NTP, 1µM of the respective primer set and 1,5 U of the Taq polymerase (Cetus, FRG). The components were prepared in a mixture, the DNA and the Taq polymerase were added thereafter. The mixture was overlaid with several drops mineral oil to prevent evaporation and incubated for 5 min at 94°C for DNA denaturation. Forty cycles of amplification were performed using a PCR processor (Coy, Ann Arbor, Michigan). Each cycle consisted of a denaturation step to 94°C of 30 sec, an annealing step to 37°C of 40 sec and an elongation step to 72°C of 60 sec. The last cycle was followed by a final step prolongation at 72°C for 7 min. Finally 20µl of the reaction mixture were analyzed by 2% agarose gel electrophoresis stained with ethidium bromide. Southern tranfer and hybridization under stringent conditions (TM -20°C) were carried out as described above. The size of the amplification products was determined by comparison with the Hae-III-restriction fragments of ΦX-174-RF-DNA.

Table 1: Sequences and locations of oligonucleotide primers in the HPV genomes

Primer	Sequence (5' to 3')	Region and nucleotide localization	Amplimer length (bp)
HPV 11-1	GGA/ATA/CAT/GCG/CCA/TGT/GG	L1 6841-6860	360
HPV 11-2	CGA/GCA/GAC/GTC/CGT/CCT/CG	L1 7181-7200	
HPV 16-1	TCA/AAA/GCC/ACT/GTG/TCC/TG	E6 421-440	120
HPV 16-2	CGT/GTT/CTT/GAT/GAT/CTG/CA	E6 521-540	
HPV 18-1	CAG/TAT/ACC/CCA/TGC/TGC/ATG/CC	E6 278-300	160
HPV 18-2	CGG/TTT/CTG/GCA/CCG/CAG/GCA/CC	E6 415-437	

Control Reactions

All experiments were performed in parallel with positive and negative controls. Negative controls included reaction mixtures lacking any DNA and mixtures with human placental DNA lacking HPV-sequences. Cloned and diluted HPV-11, -16 and -18 DNA and HPV-positive lesions (in Southern blot experiments) served as positive controls. The sensitivity of the PCR was greater than 0.0002 copies HPV-DNA per cell. To avoid false positive reactions due to contamination, filter-equipped pipette tips were used and all reagents were stored in small aliquots. Different steps of the procedure were carried out in three physically separated laboratories.

Results

77 primary endometrial carcinomas were analyzed for the prevalence of HPV-DNA. 50 patients had stage I disease according to the new FIGO classification. In 11 cases the stage was II, in 15 cases III, and one patient had stage IV disease (table 2). The histologic diagnosis was adenocarcinoma in 54 patients, 19 of which were highly, 21 medium, and 14 poor differentiated. 10 patients had adenosquamous carcinoma and in 13 cases a mixed Mullerian tumor was diagnosed (table 3).

Table 2: HPV DNA in Endometrial Carcinoma (SB+PCR) FIGO Stages

FIGO stage	n	HPV negative	HPV 16	HPV x
I	50	49	1 (PCR)	-
II	11	10	-	1 (SB)
III	15	15	-	-
IV	1	-	1 (SB+PCR)	-
	77	74	2	1

Table 3: HPV DNA in Endometrial Carcinoma (SB+PCR) Histology

Histology	n	HPV negative	HPV 16	HPV x
Adeno Ca highly diff.	19	19	-	-
Adeno Ca medium diff.	21	18	2 (1PCR) (1 SB+PCR)	1 (SB)
Adeno Ca less diff.	14	14	-	-
Adeno-squamous Ca	10	10	-	-
Mullerian mixed tumor	13	13	-	-
Endometrial Ca	77	74	2	1
Myometrium normal tissue	37	37	-	-

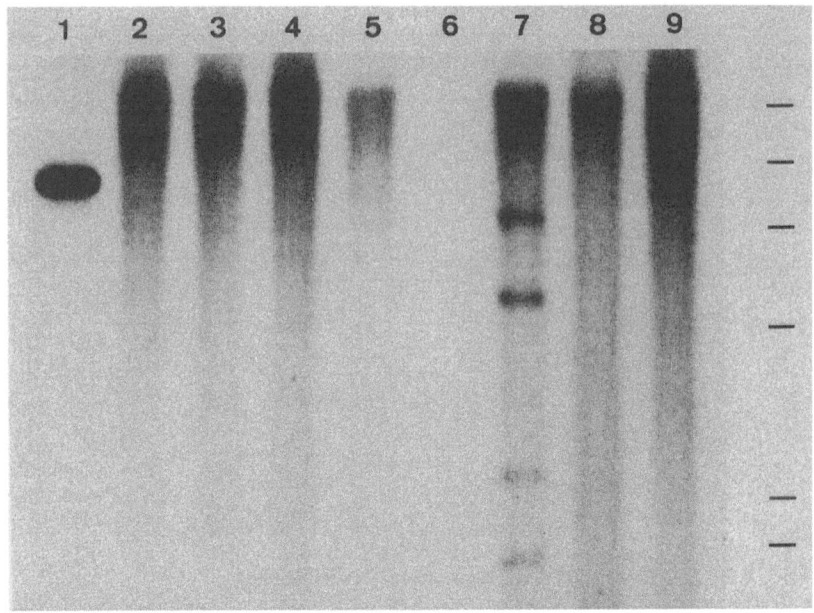

Fig. 1: Southern blot analysis of Bam HI-digested DNA from endometrial cancers. Ten µg of cellular DNA was hybridized to ^{32}P-labelled HPV-16-DNA under nonstringent conditions (Tm -35°C) and exposed for 10 days. Lane 1: reconstruction of 50 pg cloned HPV-16-DNA. Lanes 2-8: endometrial carcinoma specimens. Lane 9: human placenta. The tumor in lane 7 contained 1 cp/cg HPV-16-DNA. All detected bands were also visible after a wash under stringent conditions (Tm -20°C). Length marker phage lambda DNA/Hind III: 23.1, 9.4, 6.6, 4.4, 2.3, 2.0 kb.

HPV-DNA was detected in three of these 77 primary endometrial cancers of different histologic types (table 3) and stages (table 2) tested by Southern blot hybridization (SB) with HPV-11, -16, -18, and — in part — HPV-31 and -35 under nonstringent and stringent conditions and by polymerase chain reaction (PCR) with HPV-11-L1-, HPV-16-E6-, and HPV-18-E6-primers.

HPV-16 (1 copy/cellular genome = cp/cg) was found in the cervical tumor of a medium-differentiated endometrial adenocarcinoma stage IV (skin) in a 76-year-old patient by SB and PCR (lane 7, fig.1 and lane 5, fig. 2). The corporal tumor tissue was inadequate for DNA analysis. Primary radiation therapy was administered. A medium-differentiated adenocarcinoma in a corporal

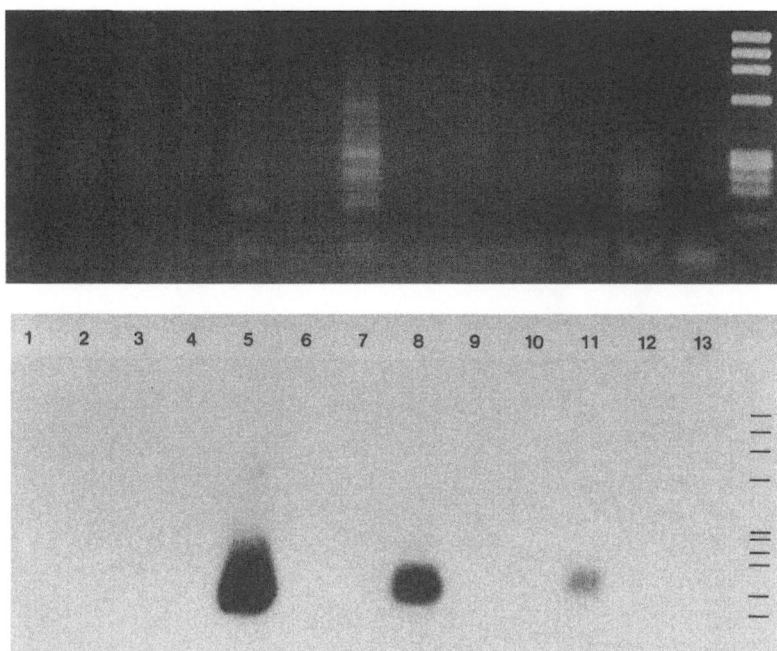

Fig. 2: Detection of HPV-16 sequences in endometrial cancer tissue by PCR.
A: Amplification products were resolved in 2% agarose gel electrophoresis. The expected 120 bp fragment is seen after ethidiumbromide staining in lanes 5, 8 and 11. Lanes 1-10: endometrial cancer specimens. Lane 11: 100 ng of HPV-16 positive cervical carcinoma DNA (1 cp/cg). Lane 12: human placenta. Lane 13: reaction without DNA template as negative control. Length marker ΦX-174-RF-DNA/Hae III: 1353, 1078, 872, 603, 310, 281/271, 234, 194, 118, 72 bp.
B: A 3-day-autoradiograph from Southern blot of gel A. The endometrial carcinomas in lanes 5 and 8 and the positive control demonstrate a signal.

curretage of endometrial carcinoma stage IB in a 93-year-old patient (also treated with primary radiation therapy) contained HPV-16 DNA (only by PCR) (lane 8, fig. 2). HPV-related sequences only hybridizing under nonstringent conditions were detected in a medium-differentiated endometrial carcinoma stage IIB in a 52 year-old patient treated by *Wertheim* hysterectomy (not shown). All three cases were estrogen- and progesterone-receptor-positive. In none of the respective cervical tissues HPV-specific histologic changes were diagnosed.

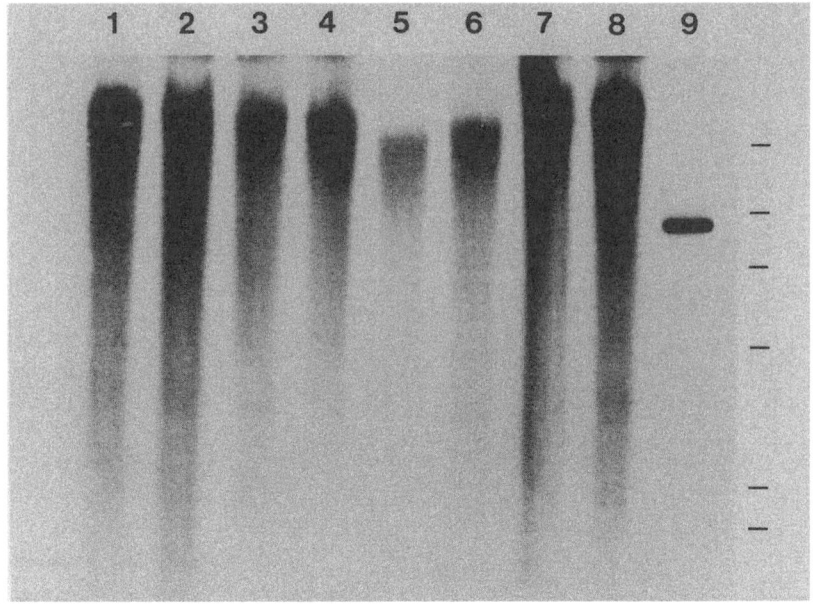

Fig. 3: Southern blot analysis of Bam HI-digested DNA from ovarian cancers. Ten μg of cellular DNA was hybridized to ^{32}p-labelled HPV-16-DNA under nonstringent conditions (Tm - 35°C). Neither after an exposition of 10 days nor after a wash under semistringent and stringent conditions and a reexposition HPV specific bands were seen. Lanes 1-7: ovarian cancer specimens. Lane 8: human placenta. Lane 9: reconstruction of 10 pg cloned HPV-16-DNA. Length marker phage lambda DNA/Hind III: 23.1, 9.4, 6.6, 4.4, 2.3, 2.0 bp.

No viral DNA was detected with the probes and primers applied in the other 74 endometrial cancer specimens, 71 of which were obtained by abdominal hysterectomy (table 3). Myometrial control tissue analyzed in 37 cases was HPV-negative.

18 ovarian cancers (pelvic and abdominal tumors) were tested for the presence of HPV-DNA under the conditions outlined above. 13 of the tumors were primary disease stage III, two stage IV, two metastases of stomach cancer and one was a recurrence of ovarian carcinoma. The histology of the primary ovarian lesions was papillary-serous in 13 cases, clear cell in one and endometrioid in one case. In none of these tumors HPV-sequences could be detected.

Discussion

Only three of 77 primary endometrial cancers and none of 18 ovarian cancers analyzed by two different DNA detection techniques in parallel contained human papillomavirus DNA. Beside the Southern blot hybridization with its high reliability and a sensitivity of 0,1 to 0,2 copies of viral DNA per cellular genome regarded as the gold standard of hybridization assays [9], we applied the polymerase chain reaction (PCR). The PCR, first described in 1985 by Saiki et al [23], has rapidly gained increasing attention by its enormous sensitivity, theoretically allowing the detection of one single target molecule in an assay. This advantage is inherently linked with serious contamination hazards.

The low detection rate of papillomavirus DNA in endometrial and ovarian cancers in contrast to cervical neoplasms is in line with the diverging epidemiological findings in these cancers [reviews: 22,17,18]. The only defined HPV-type identified in our study was HPV-16, which is also by far the most prevalent type in genital squamous carcinomas [3, review see 10]. This is in some contrast to the relatively higher prevalence of HPV-18 in cervical adenocarcinomas [26,27, review see 10]. All the three HPV-positive endometrial lesions were medium-differentiated adenocarcinomas of different stages. Two of the patients were old (76 and 93 years), while one was relatively young for the diagnosis of endometrial cancer (52 years). In one case the HPV-diagnosis was confirmed by Southern blot hybridization and PCR, while one case each was only positive by either method. This can be explained as follows. A tumor positive by PCR may not contain enough viral DNA for detection by Southern blot hybridization, while HPV-related sequences hybridizing only under nonstringent conditions cannot be amplified by type-specific primers with base mismatches to the targeted sequence.

Interestingly two of the three HPV-positive tissues were obtained by cervical biopsy or corporal curretage, confering a risk of contamination with nontumorous HPV-containing cervical cells. This possibility seems to be low due to the high age of the respective patients where HPV-infection of the cervix is rare [5] and because in none of the respective normal cervical tissues HPV-specific histologic changes were diagnosed. But it is remarkable that two of only five tumors, where the tissue was taken by biopsy or curretage contained HPV-DNA, while only one of 72 cases, where the specimens were taken after hysterectomy, contained HPV-related sequences. Although rare, the presence of HPV-DNA in cervical normal tissue of old women has been reported [5,24] and an extremely long persistence of papillomavirus infection is known [31]. These findings are in line with the results of previous studies to detect HPV-DNA in endometrial and ovarian cancer. HPV-DNA was only identified in endometrial tissue taken by biopsy in patients with concomitant HPV-associated cervical disease. MacNab et al [14] found HPV-16-DNA in two endometrial carcinomas and in four of seven specimens of normal myometrium applying Southern blot hybridization. Five of these patients had HPV-16-positive cervical carcinoma. Using labelled cellular DNA, de Villiers et al [4] failed to detect HPV-DNA in five endometrial carcinomas, while two of 11 normal endometria contained HPV-16. These endometrial specimens were taken by biopsy and both patients with HPV-16-positive endometrium had carcinoma in situ of the cervix. When care was taken to avoid contamination of the endometrial material by possibly HPV-containing cervical tissue (e.g. specimens taken after hysterectomy and tissue excised as far away from the isthmus as possible), no HPV-sequences were detected. With these precautions Bergeron et al [1] using Southern blot hybridization detected no HPV-DNA in seven normal, five hyperplastic, and 16 neoplastic endometria.

Up to now no association between ovarian neoplasia and HPV was demonstrated in two studies. The presence of HPV DNA in ovarian cancer was published only in one study [11] later on retracted for methodical problems [12]. No HPV-DNA was found in seven ovarian carcinomas by labelling cellular DNA [4]. 15 epithelial ovarian cancers in a more recent study tested by Southern blot and PCR were all HPV-negative [13].

Our results render a role of HPV in the development of endometrial and ovarian cancer unlikely, although an infection with HPV-types completely unrelated to those probed for cannot yet be totally ruled out. The sporadic detection of HPV-DNA in endometrial cancer tissue may be due to artificial spread from inapparent cervical HPV-infection.

References

1. Bergeron C., Shah K., Daniel R., Ferenczy A.: Search for human papillomaviruses in normal, hyperplastic and neoplastic endometria. Obstet. Gynecol. 72: 383-387, 1988
2. Boshart M., Gissmann L., Ikenberg H., Kleinhenz A., Scheurlen H., zur Hausen H.: A new type of papillomavirus-DNA, its presence in genital cancer biopsies and in cell lines derived from cervical cancer. EMBO J. 3: 1151-1157, 1984
3. Dürst M., Gissmann L., Ikenberg H., zur Hausen H.: A papillomavirus DNA from a cervical carcinoma and its prevalence in cancer biopsy samples from different geographic regions. Proc. Natl. Acad. Sci. USA 80: 3812-3815, 1983

4. de Villiers E.-M., Schneider A., Gross G., zur Hausen H.: Analysis of benign and malignant urogenital tumors for human papilloma virus infection by labeling cellular DNA. Med. Microbiol. Immunol. 174: 281-284, 1986
5. de Villiers E.-M., Schneider A., Miklaw H., Papendick U., Wagner D., Wesch H., Wahrendorf J., zur Hausen H.: Human papillomavirus infections in women with and without abnormal cervical cytology. Lancet ii, 703-706, 1987
6. Farnsworth A., Laverty C., Stoler M.H.: Human papillomavirus messenger RNA expression in adenocarcinoma in situ of the uterine cervix. Int. J. Gynecol. Pathol. 8: 321-330, 1989
7. Feinberg A.P., Vogelstein B.: A technique for radioloabelling DNA restriction endonuclease fragments to high specific activity. Anal. Biochem. 132: 6-13, 1983
8. Ferenczy A., Gelfand M.M., Tzipris F.: The cytodynamics of endometrial hyperplasia and carcinoma. A review. Ann. Pathol. 3: 189-202, 1983
9. Gissmann L., Dürst M., Oltersdorf T., von Knebel-Döberitz M.: Human papillomaviruses and cervical cancer. In: Cancer cells 5 Papillomaviruses. Eds.: Steinberg B.M., Brandsma J.L., Taichman L.B. Cold Spring Harbor Laboratory, 275-280, 1987
10. Ikenberg, H.: Human papillomavirus DNA in invasive genital carcinomas. In: Genital papillomavirus infections. Modern diagnosis and treatment. Eds.: Gross G., Jablonska S., Pfister H., Stegner H.E. Springer, Heidelberg, 87-112, 1990
11. Kaufman R.H., Bernstein J., Gordon A.N., Adam E., Kaplan A.L., Adler-Stohrtz K.: Detection of human papillomavirus DNA in advanced epithelial ovarian carcinoma. Gynecol. Oncol. 27: 340-349, 1987
12. Kaufman R.H., Adam E., Adler-Storthz K.: Absence of human papillomavirus (HPV) DNA sequences in epithelial ovarian carcinoma [letter] Gynecol. Oncol. 37: 148, 1990
13. Leake J., Woodruff J.D., Searle C., Daniel R., Shah K.V., Currie J.L.: Human papillomavirus and epithelial ovarian neoplasia. Gynecol. Oncol. 34: 268-273, 1989
14. MacNab J.C.M., Walkinshaw S.A., Cordiner J.W., Clements J.B.: Human papillomavirus in clinically and histologically normal tissue of patients with genital cancer. New Engl. J. Med. 315: 1052-1058, 1986
15. Münger K., Phelps W.C., Bubb V., Howley P., Schlegel R.: The E6 and E7 genes of human papillomavirus type 16 together are necessary and sufficient for transformation of primary human keratinocytes. J. Virol. 63: 4417-4421, 1989
16. Okagaki T., Tase T., Twiggs L.B., Carson L.T.: Histogenesis of cervical adenocarcinoma with reference to human papillomavirus 18 as a carcinogen. J. Reprod. Med. 34: 639-644, 1989
17. Parazzini F., Franceschi S., La Vecchia C., Fasoli M.: The epidemiology of ovarian cancer. Gynecol. Oncol. 43: 9-23, 1991 a
18. Parazzini F., La Vecchia C., Bocciolone L., Franceschi S.: The epidemiology of endometrial cancer. Gynecol. Oncol. 41, 1-16, 1991 b
19. Pflederer A.: Malignome des Ovars. In: Klinik der Frauenheilkunde und Geburtshilfe, Bd. 12. Eds.: Schmidt-Mathiesen H., Wulf K.H. Urban und Schwarzenberg, München, 45-129, 1989

20. Pfleiderer A.: Endometrial malignancy. Curr. Opin. Obstet. Gyn. 3: 92-99, 1991
21. Rigoni-Stern D.A.: Fatti statistici relativi alle mallattie cancerose che servirono di base alle poche cose delta dal dotte. G. Progr. Pathol. Therap. Ser. 2: 507-517, 1842
22. Rotkin I.D.: A comparison review of key epidemiological studies in cervical cancer related to current searches for transmissible agents. Cancer Res. 33: 1353-1367, 1973
23. Saiki R., Scharf S., Falcoona F., Mullis K., Han G., Erlich H., Arnheim N.: Enzymatic amplification of β-globin genomic sequences and restriction site analysis for diagniosis of siccle cell anemia. Science 230, 1350-1354, 1985
24. Schneider A., de Villiers E.-M., Schneider V.: Multifocal squamous neoplasia of the female genital tract. Significance of human papillomavirus infection in the vagina after hysterectomy. Obstet. Gynecol. 70: 294-298, 1987
25. Siiteri P.K.: Extraglandular oestrogen fraction and serum binding of oestradiol: Relationship to cancer. J. Endocrinol. 89, 119P-129P, 1981
26. Smotkin D., Berek J.S., Fu Y.S., Hacker N.F., Major F.J., Wettstein F.O.: Human papillomavirus deoxyribonucleic acid in adenocarcinoma and adenosquamous carcinoma of the uterine cervix. Obstet. Gynecol. 68: 241-244, 1986
27. Tase T., Okagaki T., Clark B.A., Manias D.A., Ostrow R.S., Twiggs L.B., Faras A.J.: Human papillomavirus types and localization in adenocarcinoma and adenosquamous carcinoma of the uterine cervix: A study by in situ DNA hybridization. Cancer Res. 48: 993-998, 1988
28. Tase T., Okagaki T., Clark B.A., Twiggs L.B., Ostrow R.S., Faras A.J.: Human papillomavirus DNA in glandular dysplasia and microglandular hyperplasia: presumed precursors of adenocarcinoma of the uterine cervix. Obstet. Gynecol. 73: 1005-1008, 1989
29. Wagner D., Ikenberg H., Böhm N., Gissmann L.: Type specific identification of human papillomavirus in cervical smears by DNA in situ hybridization. Obstet. Gynecol. 62: 767-772, 1984
30. zur Hausen H., Schneider A.: The role of papillomaviruses in human anogenital cancer. In: The Papovaviridiae 2. Eds.: Salzman N.P., Howley P.M. Plenum Press, New York and London, 245-263, 1987 b
31. zur Hausen H.: Human papillomaviruses in the pathogenesis of anogenital cancer. Virology 184: 9-13, 1991

Acknowledgements: The authors thank Dr. L. Gissmann who provided the cloned HPV-11, -16 and -18-DNA and Dr. A. Lorincz for the DNA of HPV-31 and -35.
This work was supported by the Deutsche Forschungsgemeinschaft Ik 1-1/1.

Zur Immunhistologie des Dysgerminoms

J. Dietl, H.-P. Horny, E. Kaiserling

Die Mikroarchitektur des Dysgerminoms wird typischerweise von einer dichten zellulären Stromareaktion bestimmt, welche auf eine aktive Immunantwort gegenüber den Tumorzellen hinweist. Während bei dem wesentlich häufigeren Seminom eine immunhistologische Charakterisierung der tumorinfiltrierenden lymphoretikulären Zellen (TIL) bereits erfolgte [1], wurde das Dysgerminom des Ovars dahingehend noch nicht untersucht.

Material und Methode

Paraffineingebettetes Material von 3 Dysgerminomen wurde verwendet, in einem Fall stand auch kryokonserviertes Gewebe zur Verfügung. Die 5µm dikken Schnitte wurden mit HE, PAS, Giemsa und Gömöri's Silber gefärbt. Die immunhistologischen Färbungen wurden nach der Methode von Hsu et al. [5] durchgeführt. Die verwendeten monoklonalen Antikörper sind in der Tabelle aufgeführt.

Ergebnisse (Tabelle)

Alle drei Fälle zeigten das typische histologische Bild eines Dysgerminoms, bestehend aus Nestern und Strängen großer polygonaler Tumorzellen mit hellem Zytoplasma und prominenten Nukleoli, umgeben von fibrovaskulären Septen mit einer ausgeprägten zellulären Stromareaktion. Die immunhistologische Untersuchung ergab, daß die Tumorzellen im allgemeinen nicht mit den angewandten hämopoetischen und nicht-hämopoetischen Antikörpern reagierten, insbesondere exprimierten sie keine HLA-Klasse II-Antigene. In einem Fall (Nr. 3) zeigte eine geringe Anzahl von Tumorzellen eine positive Reaktion mit den T-Zell-assoziierten Antikörpern UCHL 1 und DF-T1 und mit dem Makrophagen-Marker KP1.

Tabelle 1: Antikörper und immunhistologische Befunde beim Dysgerminom

Antikörper	Reaktivität/Spezifität	Fall 1 TU	Fall 1 TIL	Fall 2 TU	Fall 2 TIL	Fall 3 TU	Fall 3 TIL
UCHL1 (CD45RO), A	T Zell-assoziiertes Antigen	0	++	?	+++	(+)	+++
DF-T1 (CD43), A	T Zell-assoziiertes Antigen	0	+++	?	+/++	(+)	+++
L26 (CD20), A	B Zell-assoziiertes Antigen	0	+++	0	+	0	+/++
Ki-B3, B	B Zell-assoziiertes Antigen	0	+/++	0	(+)	0	+/++
Leu-7 (CD57), C	NK-Zellen	0	+/++	0	0	0	(+)/+
KP1 (CD68), A	Monozyten/Makrophagen-assoziiertes Antigen	+	++	?	++	(+)	+++
Anti-S100 Protein (CD1), A	T immun-akzessorische Zelle	?	++	?	+	?	(+)
MAC387, A	Makrophagen, epithel.Zellen	?	+++	?	+++	?	+++
Ber-H2 (CD30), A	Hodgkin Zell-assoz. Antigen	0	(+)	0	0	0	(+)
DAKO-M746, A	HLA-DR/2	0	++	0	+/++	?	+++
Anti-Vimentin, A	Mesenchymale Zellen	0	0	0	0	0	0
KL1, D	Pancytokeratin	(+)	0	0	0	(+)	0
F VIII Antigen, A	Endotheliale Zellen	0	0	0	0	0	0
Anti-α-Fetoprot., A	α-Fetoprotein	0	0	0	0	0	0
Anti-CEA, A	Carcino-embryonales Antigen	?	0	0	0	0	0
T3 (CD3), A	CD3/T3 Komplex	0	+++	n.d.		n.d.	
T4 (CD4), A	Helper/inducer T Zellen	0	+/++	n.d.		n.d.	
T8 (CD8), A	Suppressor/zytotox.T Zellen	0	+++/++	n.d.		n.d.	
T6 (CD1), A	Thymozyten/dendrit.Zellen	0	(+)	n.d.		n.d.	
βF1, E	β Kette des T Zellrezeptors	0	+++	n.d.		n.d.	
BMA031, F	α/β Heterodimer des T Zellrezeptors	0	++/+++	n.d.		n.d.	
TCRδ1, E	δKette des γ/δ Heterodimer des T Zellrezeptors	0	(+)/+	n.d.		n.d.	
Leu 19 (CD56), C	NK-Zellen (NHK1)	0	(+)/+	n.d.		n.d.	
IL-2R (CD25), E	Interleukin-2 Rezeptor	0	+/++	n.d.		n.d.	
DAKO-TfR, A	Transferrin-Rezeptor	0	++	n.d.		n.d.	

TU = Tumorzellen; TIL = tumorinfiltrierende lymphoretikuläre Zellen, wie Lymphozyten und epithelioide Zellen; n.d. = nicht durchgeführt; A = DAKO, Hamburg; B = Feller et al. [3]; C = Becton Dickinson, Heidelberg; D = Dianova, Hamburg; E = T Cell Sciences, Cambridge, MA; F = Behring-Werke, Marburg; 0 = negativ; (+) = sehr wenig gefärbte Zellen; + = wenig gefärbte Zellen; ++ = mäßig viele gefärbte Zellen; +++ = sehr viele gefärbte Zellen; ? =nicht bestimmbar

Die TIL bestanden zum ganz überwiegenden Teil aus T-Zellen (CD43+, CD45R0+), epithelioiden Zellen/Histiozyten und Riesenzellen (MAC 387+, CD 68+), während B-Zellen (CD 20+, Ki-B3+) und NK-Zellen (CD 56+, CD 57+) nicht oder nur sehr wenige anzutreffen waren.

An dem kryokonservierten Gewebe konnte nachgewiesen werden, daß die meisten der intratumoralen T-Zellen den α/β-T-Zellrezeptor exprimierten, während γ/δ+ T-Zellen extrem selten auftraten. Die meisten der intratumoralen T-Zellen gehörten zu dem CD 8+ (zytotoxisch/suppressor) Subtyp.

Diskussion

Die immunhistologische Phänotypisierung der TIL im Dysgerminom ergab, daß die Mehrzahl der Zellen aus T-Lymphozyten und epithelioiden Zellen bestand, während B-Lymphozyten und NK-Zellen kaum anzutreffen waren. Diese Dominanz der T-Zellen und Histiozyten wurde auch in anderen malignen Tumoren gefunden [2,4]. Die Gegenwart nur weniger CD 56+ und CD 57+ NK-Zellen in Dysgerminomen steht in Übereinstimmung mit Befunden beim Seminom [1]. Die Verteilung der α/β- und γ/δ-Heterodimere des T-Zellantigenrezeptors ergibt für die überwiegende Mehrzahl der TIL den Phänotyp: CD 3+, α/β+, γ/δ-.

Da an den Tumorzellen des Dysgerminoms keine HLA-Klasse II-Antigene nachgewiesen werden konnten, ist die Akkumulation von T-Zellen und Histiozyten offensichtlich unabhängig von der Expression der MHC-Antigene an den neoplastischen Zellen. Üblicherweise erkennen T-Lymphozyten Antigene über den T-Zellrezeptor nur in enger topographischer Assoziation mit Klasse I oder II-MHC-Produkten (MHC-Restriktion der T-Zellerkennung).

Überraschenderweise reagierte in einem Fall eine kleine Anzahl von Tumorzellen mit den beiden T-Zell assoziierten Antikörpern UCHL 1 und DF-T1 und mit dem Makrophagenmarker KP1. Bei dieser Patientin konnten auch histologisch positive paraaortale Lymphknoten nachgewiesen werden. Es bleibt Spekulation, ob diese ungewöhnliche Marker-Expression in einer Beziehung zur Progression und Disseminierung solcher Tumoren steht.

Literatur

1. Bell D.A, Flotte T.J., Bhan A.K.: Immunhistochemical characterization of seminoma and its inflammatory cell infiltrate. Hum. Pathol. 18: 511-520, 1987
2. Dietl J., Horny H.-P., Buchholz F.: Lymphoreticular cells in invasive carcinoma of the uterine cervix. An immunohistological study. Int. J. Obstet. Gynecol. 34: 179-182, 1991
3. Feller A.C., Wacker H.H., Moldenhauer G., Radzun H.-J., Parwaresch M.R.: Monoclonal antibody KiB3 detects a formalin resistant antigen on normal and neoplastic B cells. Blood 70: 629-636, 1987
4. Horst H.-A., Horny H.-P.: Characterization and frequency distribution of lymphoreticular infiltrates in axillary lymph node metastases of invasive ductal carcinoma of the breast. Cancer 60: 3001-3007, 1987
5. Hsu S.M., Raine L., Fanger H.: Use of avidin-biotin-peroxidase complex (ABC) in immunoperoxidase techniques. J. Histochem. Cytochem. 29: 577-580, 1981

Modulation von tumor-assoziierten Antigenen durch Cholesterylhemisuccinat bei Ovarialkarzinom-Zellen

Th. Neßelhut, A. Perschl, R. Dietrich, W. Kuhn

Zusammenfassung

There is strong evidence that malignant cells bear tumor-associated antigens (TAA). The antigenicity of tumor cells, however, is too weak to elicit an effective immune reaction against tumor growth. In order to induce an increase of the immunogenicity, ovarian carcinoma cells growing in cell culture were treated with cholesteryl hemisuccinate (CHS). This agent is well known as a modulator of the fluidity of the cell membrane causing an altered expression of a variety of membrane proteins, possibly by vertical displacement. Antibodies detecting these cells were found by immunocytochemistry in autologous and allogenic ascites. Using flow cytometry analysis, an increase in fluorescence intensity was observed on trypsinized cells stained with purified autologous and allogenic IgG after CHS incubation for 2 to 3 h. Avoiding possible trypsin induced shedding of antigens, a cell ELISA was developed to analyse the exposition of antigens on viable adherent cells in 96-well plates. Using this approach, the kinetic of the autologous and allogenic antibody bindings could be studied. These experiments confirmed the results obtained by flow cytometry in respect to the autologous antibody binding. The binding of allogenic IgG was in this case far less enhanced by CHS. The results suggest a potent role of CHS as an enhancer of antigen exposition. Therefore, CHS could be a possible candidate for an immunomodulating agent for using in an active specific vaccination and immunotherapy of cancer.

Einleitung

Der Einsatz monoklonaler Antikörper in der Tumorimmunologie hat zur Identifikation und Charakterisierung zahlreicher humaner Tumorassoziierter Antigene (TAA) geführt. Die Definition dieser TAA ist nach wie vor umstritten. Ng et al. [4] definieren TAA als Antigene, die auf gesunden Gegenstücken einer Tumorzelle nicht exprimiert werden. Order et al. [5] bezeichnen TAA als normale Gewebsproteine, deren Konzentrationen aufgrund des Krebsgeschehens ansteigen, während nach Levine [2] TAA Zellproteine darstellen, die eine Immunantwort im Wirt hervorrufen können.

In Modellsystemen erwiesen sich einige TAA als geeignete Ziele für unterschiedliche immunologische Reaktionen. Eliminierung von Tumorzellen durch immunologische Reaktionen konnten von Casellas et al. [1] und Pendurthi et al. [6] nachgewiesen werden. Jedoch ist die Antigenität der meisten Tumoren so gering, daß Karzinome in der Regel trotz des Evozierens von Immunreaktionen weiter wachsen können. Therapeutisch könnte eine Verstärkung der Tumorantigenität von Nutzen sein.

Hier setzt die vorliegende Arbeit an. Es soll anhand von in vitro Experimenten gezeigt werden, daß durch die Inkubation mit zellmembranwirksamen Substanzen die Antigenität von Ovarialkarzinom-Zellen erheblich gesteigert werden kann. Modellhaft soll dies mit der Cholesterylhemisuccinat-Wirkung demonstriert werden. Auf der Basis dieser Exprimente ist ein methodischer Ansatz zur Herstellung von hochpotenten Tumorvakzinen gegeben.

Material und Methoden

Präparation von Ovarialkarzinomzellen aus Aszites
Frischer, unter sterilen Bedingungen entnommener Aszites wurde für 10 min bei 200 x g zentrifugiert. Der Überstand wurde zur Präparation von IgG entnommen und die im Sediment befindlichen Zellen in wenig Aszites aufgenommen. Diese Zellsuspension wurde zur Isolierung von Tumorzellen einer Zentrifugation bei 200 x g für 30 min. im Dichtegradienten unterzogen, der aus einer 60% Percoll-Lösung bestand. Die Tumorzellen, die sich in der Interphase befanden, wurden in RPMI-Zellkulturmedium überführt, das 10% fetales Kälberserum, Penicillin und Streptomycin enthielt. Nach einer weiteren Zentrifugation bei 200 x g für 10 min. wurden die im Sediment befindlichen Zellen in das o.g. Zellkulturmedium überführt und in Kulturflaschen im Brutschrank angezogen.

Zell-ELISA
Die Ovarialkarzinomzellen wurden durch eine Trypsinbehandlung von den Zellkulturflaschen abgelöst und nach Waschen in Zellkulturmedium auf eine Zellzahl von 50.000 Zellen/ml eingestellt. Jeweils 200 µl dieser Zellsuspension wurde pro Napf auf eine 96-Well-Rundboden-Mikrotiterplatte aufgetragen und die Zellen 36 Stunden im Brutschrank kultiviert. Nach dem Dekantieren des Kulturmediums und Waschen wurden die Ovarialkarzinomzellen mit

einer CHS/PVP-Lösung für 3 h im Brutschrank belassen. Nach zweimaligem Waschen mit PBS wurde mit aus Aszites angereichertem IgG, das in PBS gelöst war, in einem Volumen von 200 µl/Napf für 2 h inkubiert. Das an die Tumorzellen gebundene IgG wurde nach zweimaligem Waschen mit Kulturmedium mit Biotin konjugiertem antihumeanem IgG aus Ziege in einer Verdünnung von 1:100 für 90 min zur Reaktion gebracht. Nach gründlichem Waschen erfolgte eine einstündige Inkubation mit Streptavidin-Peroxidase-Lösung, die in einer Verdünnung von 1:100 zur Anwendung kam. Abschließend wurde pro Napf 125 µl Farb/Substratlösung hinzugegeben, die aus 3% H_2O_2 ABTS bestand. Die Extinktion des entwickelten Farbstoffs wurde im Plattenphotometer der Firma SLT, Österreich, auf 96-Well-Flachboden-Mikrotiterplatten gemessen.

Anreicherung von IgG aus Aszites
IgG wurde über eine Protein-G-Affinitäts-Chromatographie-Säule von der Firma Pharmacia nach Angaben des Herstellers isoliert.

SDS-Polyacrylamid-Gelelektrophorese und Western-Blot
Beide Methoden sind bei Neßelhut et al. [3] beschrieben.

Ergebnisse

Die Zellproteine, die von Ovarialkarzinomzellen spontan in das Kulturmedium abgegeben wurden oder die sich durch Detergenzbehandlung (CHAPS) ablösen ließen, wurden elektrophoretisch aufgetrennt und im Western-Blot in Hinblick auf das Bindungsverhalten mit IgG aus Patientinnenseren getestet. Wie die Abb. 1 zeigt, reagierten verschiedene Proteinbanden sowohl mit allogenen als autologen IgG-Antikörpern.

Auf fixierten Ovarialkarzinomzellen konnte unter Einsatz von FITC-gekoppelten gegen humanes IgG gerichteten Antikörpern die Bindung von autologen und allogenen Antikörpern in zytologischen Präparaten gleichfalls nachgewiesen werden (ohne Abb.).

Das Bindungsverhalten von autologen und allogenen IgG-Antikörpern wurde im Zell-ELISA in kinetischen Studien untersucht. Es zeigte sich, daß ein träges Reaktionsverhalten bei unbehandelten Ovarialkarzinomzellen sowohl gegenüber allogenen als auch autologen Antikörpern typisch war (Abb. 2 u. 3). Eine wesentliche Steigerung der IgG-Bindung konnte mit CHS erzielt werden. Dieser Effekt war am stärksten im autologen System ausgeprägt (Abb. 2-4).

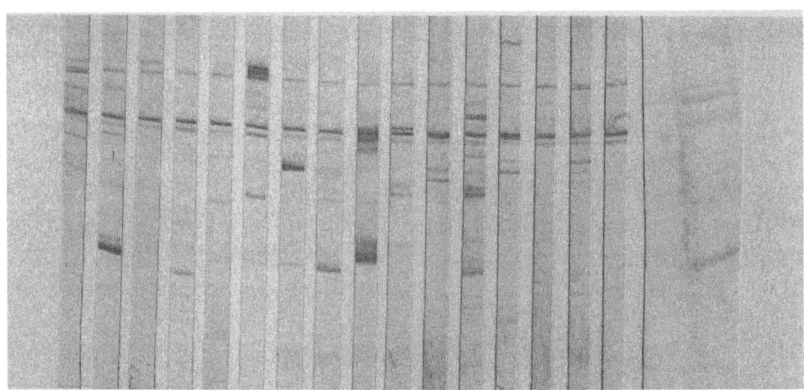

Abb. 1: Western-Blot von Ovarialkarzinom-Zellkulturüberstand nach Detergenzbehandlung mit Patientinnenseren inkubiert. Gebundenes IgG wurde mit antihumanem IgG Antikörper nachgewiesen.

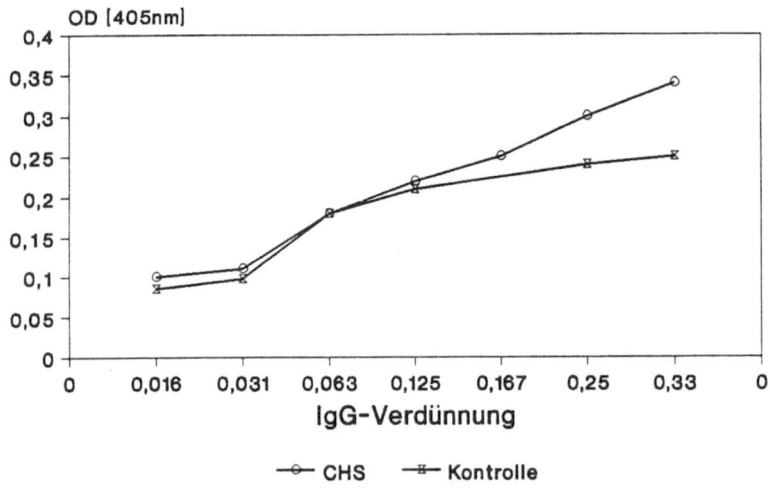

Abb.2: Bindungskinetik von allogenen IgG-Antikörpern und humane Ovarialkarzinom-Zellen im Zell-ELISA

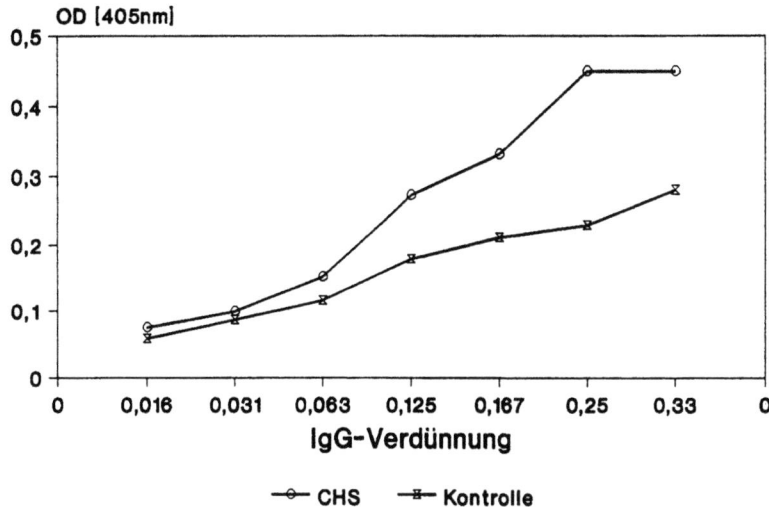

Abb. 3: Bindungskinetik von autologen IgG-Antikörpern und humanen Ovarialkarzinomzellen im Zell-ELISA

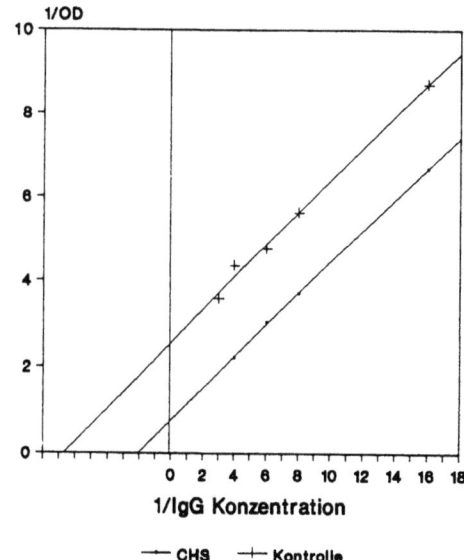

Abb. 4: Gleiche Daten wie in Abb. 3, doppeltreziprok aufgetragen.

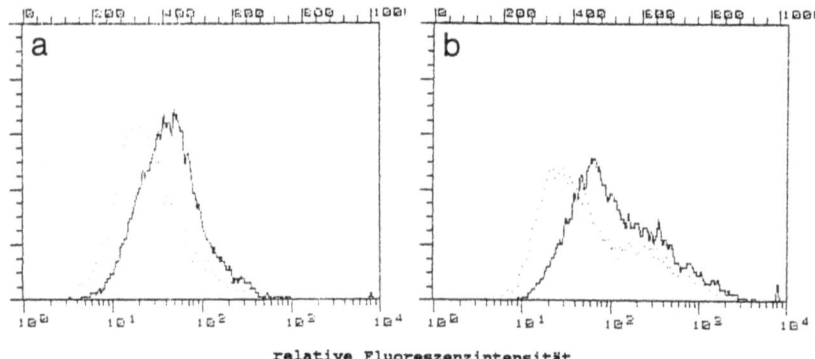

Abb. 5: Bindungsverhalten von allogenem (a) und autologem (b) IgG an Ovarialkarzinomzellen in der Durchflußzytometrie. Linke Kurve: Unbehandelte Zellen. Rechte Kurve: CHS-behandelte Zellen

Die Durchflußzytometrie bestätigte diesen Befund, indem nach CHS-Behandlung von Ovarialkarzinomzellen und Inkubation mit autologem und allogenem IgG eine deutliche Signalverstärkung mit einer Rechtsverschiebung der Markierungskurve nachweisbar war (Abb. 5).

Schlußfolgerungen

1. Ovarialkarzinomzellen bilden Proteine, die durch Detergens von den Zellen abgelöst werden und an IgG aus Patientinnenseren binden können.

2. Die Behandlung von Ovarialkarzinomzellen in vitro mit CHS führt zu einer verstärkten Exposition der Tumorantigene.

3. Die Ergebnisse zeigen, daß aus CHS-behandelten Ovarialkarzinomzellen Onkolysate hergestellt werden können, bei deren Anwendung eine verstärkte Immunreaktion in Ovarialkarzinom-Patientinnen zu erwarten ist.

Literatur

1. Casellas P. et al.: Int. J. Cancer 30: 437, 1982
2. Levine A.J.: Adv. Cancer Res. 37: 75, 1982
3. Neßelhut et al.: Arch. Gynecol. Obstet. 246: 97, 1989
4. Ng et al.: Adv. Intern. Med. 28: 253, 1983
5. Order et al.: Int. J. Radiat. Oncol. Biol. Phys. 8: 259, 1982
6. Pendurithi et al.: Int. J. Cancer 46: 1021, 1990

II. Tumorausbreitung und Prognosefaktoren

Die intra- und retroperitoneale Ausbreitung des Ovarialkarzinoms

H. Pickel

Der Beginn der neoplastischen Umwandlung des Keimepithels sowohl an der Ovarialoberfläche, als auch in den Einschlußzysten ist nie mit hinreichender Sicherheit belegt worden. Weitgehend gesichert erscheint jedoch die Zellsegregation aus dem karzinomatös veränderten Ovar. Sie geht zum einen durch die Exfoliation aus oberflächlich entwickelten papillären Tumorformationen vor sich und zum anderen ist die Penetration von Karzinomzellen durch die Tumorkapsel von Zysten, die von Geschwulstformationen erfüllt sind, ein durchaus denkbarer Propagationsmodus. Es ist allerdings nicht bekannt, ab welcher kritischen Tumorgröße diese Vorgänge wirksam werden. Die abgelösten Tumorzellen sammeln sich primär caudalwärts im Cavum Douglasii und setzen sich am Peritoneum parietale des kleinen Beckens sowie am Peritoneum viscerale der pelvinen Nachbarorgane wie Uterus und Rectum fest. Auf diese Weise kann es zur Ausbildung ausgedehnter krebsiger Rasen, aber auch knolliger Tumormassen im kleinen Becken kommen. Mit einer bilateralen Kanzerisierung der Ovarien ist zu rechnen. Sie ist in einem Drittel aller Fälle zu beobachten [4,9]. Das kontralaterale Ovar kann bereits in den frühen Stadien der Karzinomentwicklung (Stadium Ia 17,5%) metastatisch besiedelt werden [9].

Die weitere Ausbreitung abgeschilferter Karzinomzellen erfolgt mit dem Strom der Peritonealflüssigkeit in die Abdominalhöhle. Die mobilen Geschwulstzellen werden auf dem Peritoneum viscerale und parietale implantiert. Hierbei spielen immunologische Vorgänge zwischen Tumorzellen und den Peritonealdeckzellen mit, die über das Angehen der Metastasierung entscheiden. Durch den negativen hydrostatischen Druck gefördert, kommt es zur Tumorzellmigration cranialwärts, vor allem in den rechtsseitigen diaphragmalen Raum [2]. Desweiteren werden die Oberflächen vor allem des rechten Leberlappens und der Milz, sowie das Omentum majus metastatisch besiedelt [17]. Im Zuge der Metastasierung am Peritoneum des Zwerchfells dringen Tumorzellen in die abführenden und perforierenden diaphragmalen Lymphgefäße ein und verlegen so den lymphatischen Abstrom. Damit ist die Pathogenese des Ascites zumindest teilweise zu erklären. Bei Weiterleitung einer krebsigen Thromboembolie der diaphragmalen Lymphgefäße kommt es zur breitflächi-

Tabelle 1: Intraabdominelle Tumorausbreitung bei 234 Frauen mit operierten Ovarialkarzinomen der Stadien III und IV

Stadium	n	oberflächliche Lebermetastasen	peritoneale Carcinomatose	isolierte Omentum metastasen	intrahepatische Metastasen
III	190	30 (16%)	136 (72%)	88 (46%)	0
IV	44	24 (55%)	30 (68%)	4 (9%)	19 (43%)
Gesamt	234	54	166	92	19

gen Metastasierung in den Pleuraraum und damit zur Carcinosis pleurae. Autoptische Studien bei Patienten, die am Ovarialkarzinom verstorben sind, haben ergeben, daß die Tumorabsiedelung am parietalen Peritoneum in 83% und am Dick- und Dünndarm in 50% bzw. 44% zu finden ist [13]. Eigene Untersuchungen haben ergeben, daß das Maximum der abdominellen Metastasierung im Spätstadium des Ovarialkarzinoms im Oberbauch konzentriert ist, der bekanntlich auch eine Prädilektionsstelle für die Tumorrezidivierung darstellt. Im Stadium III wurden nur bei 16%, im Stadium IV hingegen bei 55% der Patienten Metastasen am Peritoneum der Leberoberfläche gefunden. Die ausgedehnte Peritonealkarzinose hingegen wurde im Stadium III und IV mit 72% zu 68% etwa gleich häufig festgestellt [10]. Merkwürdig ist hingegen, daß das große Netz im Stadium III wohl in 46%, im Stadium IV aber nur in 9% der Fälle metastatisch ergriffen war [10] (Tabelle 1).

Eine operationstechnisch besonders wichtige intraabdominelle Lokalisation der Peritonealkarzinose ist der Gastrointestinaltrakt. WU et al. [17] haben drei intraabdominelle Metastasierungstypen beschrieben: Im ersten Fall fanden sich multiple, feinknotige und oberflächlich gelegene Absiedelungen, die die Hauptmasse, nämlich 81%, der peritonealen Dünndarmmetastasen stellten. Der zweite, seltenere, intestinale Metastasierungstyp zeichnete sich durch eine Tumorinfiltration vor allem des Mesenterium aus. Dadurch wird der Dünndarm mit dem zugehörigen Mesenterium so stark zusammengezogen, daß ein starres Konvolut entsteht.

Am häufigsten war der dritte Metastasierungstyp, der in 95% der Fälle zu einer großflächigen und grobknotigen Peritonealkarzinose vor allem des Sigma und des Rectums führt. Das Endresultat sind große, schwer resezierbare, mit intestinaler Obstruktion einhergehende Konglomerattumoren im Rectum-Sigma-Bereich. Die Ausbreitung des Ovarialkarzinoms über die Peritonealoberfläche muß aber nicht nur durch Implantationsmetastasen erfolgen. Es gibt auch eine multifokale Geschwulstentstehung auf dem Peritoneum, wobei diese Tumoren histopathologisch von echten Ovarialkarzinommetastasen nicht zu unterscheiden sind. Es wird diskutiert, ob diese Neoplasien zumindest im Peritoneum des kleinen Beckens nicht aus restierendem embryonalem Coelomepithel, welches sich dort in sogenanntes Müller'sches Gangepithel mit maligner Determinierung umwandelt, entstehen können [1,15].

Schon sehr kleine Malignome geben nach Überwindung lokaler immunologischer und mechnischer Barrieren Tumorzellen in das lymphatische Gefäßsystem ab. Wie bei anderen Malignomen vollzieht sich der Transport der Tumorzellen im Gefäßsystem bevorzugt auf lymphatischem Wege. Zahlreiche abführende kleine Lymphgefäße aus dem Ovar vereinigen sich im Hilus ovarii und bilden dort einen Lymphgefäßplexus. Von diesem subovariellen Plexus gehen in der Hauptsache drei verschiedene Routen für den Lymphabstrom aus [3,9,11]: Zum einen gehen aus dem subovariellen Plexus 6-8 Lymphgefäße hervor, die die ovariellen Blutgefäße begleiten und in die paraaortalen Lymphknoten zwischen der Aortenbifurkation und dem Diaphragma münden. Dieser Lymphabfluß wurde bislang als der wichtigste angesehen [2,14]. Ein anderer Lymphabfluß geht gleichfalls vom subovariellen Plexus im Hilus ovarii aus, wird aber über das Ligamentum latum zu den obturatorischen Lymphknoten geführt [11]. Diese Knoten sind durch eine Reihe von anastomosierenden Lymphgefäßen mit den externa iliacalen sowie medialen und lateralen tiefen iliacalen Lymphknoten, aber auch mit den paraaortalen Lymphknoten verknüpft [3,11]. Eine dritte, klinisch allerdings weniger bedeutsame, Route für den Lymphabstrom geht entlang der Ligamenta rotunda in die externen iliacalen aber auch inguinalen Lymphknoten [9,11]. Demnach sind alle retroperitonealen Lymphknotenstationen, die die Lymphflüssigkeit aus den Ovarien aufnehmen, zumindestens bis zur Aortenbifurkation miteinander vernetzt, sodaß eine große Variationsbreite für die lymphatische Tumorausbreitung bzw. Metastasierung im kleinen Becken gegeben ist. Autoptische Studien ergaben ein uneinheitliches Frequenzmuster hinsichtlich der Metastasierung in die retroperitonealen Knoten. Bergman stellte bei 80% seiner untersuchten Fälle Metastasen in den pelvinen und in 78% Absiedelungen in den paraaortalen Lymphknoten fest [9]. Rose et al. [13] fanden in ihrem Obduktionsgut in 48% pelvine und in 58% der Fälle paraaortale Lymphknotenmetastasen. Zum Unterschied vom Lymphknoten-Sampling haben klinische Untersuchungen auf Grund von systematischen retroperitonealen Lymphadenektomien gezeigt, daß die Metastasenfrequenz in die pelvinen Lymphknoten etwas höher lag als die in den paraaortalen Lymphknoten (Tabelle 2).

Tabelle 2: Metastatischer Befall der retroperitonealen Lymphknoten im Stadium III

	Prozentsatz mit pos. pelvinen Knoten	Prozentsatz mit pos. paraaortalen Knoten	Art der Lymphadenektomie
Averette et al. 1983	36	41	sampling
Chen & Lee 1983	13	42	sampling
Graz 1990	71	67	systematisch
Wu et al. 1989	64	38	systematisch

Die Angaben in der Tabelle 2 könnten den Schluß zulassen, daß die metastatische Besiedlung in der pelvinen und paraaortalen Lymphknotenregion simultan erfolgt und daß der alleinige Befall der pelvinen oder paraaortalen Knoten nur selten vorkommt. Daß diese Annahme nicht zutrifft, zeigt die Tabelle 3. Bezieht man sich nur auf die positiven Fälle, so wurde der gleichzeitige Befall bei Wu et al. [17] in 28% und bei Burghardt et al. [5] in 38% der Fälle gefunden. Dementsprechend fand sich der alleinige Befall der pelvinen Knoten in 19 bzw. 10% und der alleinige Befall der paraaortalen Knoten in jeweils 10%. Bei systematischer Lymphadenektomie ist ein Anstieg der Metastasenfrequenz in den retroperitonealen, besonders der pelvinen Lymphknoten mit zunehmendem Tumorstadium zu beobachten [5,10,17]. Bei Nachweis positiver Lymphknoten gehört der Fall dem FIGO-Stadium IIIc an. Werden die Stadien aber nur nach dem intraabdominalen Befund gewertet, so findet man, daß bereits bei Patienten im Stadium I Lymphknotenmetastasen vorkommen können. Im Stadium II verdoppelt sich die Metastasenfrequenz bereits, um im Stadium III eine Häufigkeit von mehr als 70% zu erreichen. Die Metastasenfrequenz in den pelvinen Lymphknoten über alle Stadien betrug 62%. WU et al. [17] gelangte 1989 zu fast identischen Ergebnissen (58%)(Tabelle 4).

Auch innerhalb der Subgruppen des Stadiums III ist ein Frequenzanstieg der Lymphknotenmetastasen nachzuweisen (Tabelle 5). Man sieht, daß die Metastasenfrequenz im Stadium IIIa etwa derjenigen im Stadium II entspricht, während sie im Stadium IIIc das gewaltige Ausmaß von fast 83% erreicht. Hinsichtlich der absoluten Zahl an metastatisch befallenen Lymphknoten pro Fall wiesen zumeist ein bis zwei Knoten Karzinomabsiedelungen auf. Es gab aber auch Fälle, bei denen Metastasen in bis zu 44 Lymphdrüsen nachgewiesen wurden.

Tabelle 3: Metastasenbefall der pelvinen und paraaortalen Lymphknoten bei Patienten mit systematischer Lymphadenektomie

Lymphknoten (pelvin/paraaortal)	Wu et al. 1989		Burghardt et al. 1991	
	n	% mit pos. Knoten	n	% mit pos. Knoten
positiv/positiv	19	28	46	38
positiv/negativ	13	19	13	10
negativ/positiv	7	10	10	10
negativ/negativ	30	-	36	-
Gesamt	69		105	

Tabelle 4: Frequenz der Lymphknotenmetastasen und intraabdominelles Tumorstadium

Stadium	Burghardt et al. 1991			Wu et al. 1989		
	n	Pat. mit pos. Knoten		n	Pat. mit pos. Knoten	
I	37	9	(24%)	7	1	(14%)
II	14	7	(50%)	8	3	(38%)
III	114	84	(74%)	59	38	(64%)
IV	15	11	(73%)	3	3	(100%)
Gesamt	180	111	(63%)	77	45	(58%)

Tabelle 5: Peliviner Lymphknotenbefall in den Substadien des Stadiums III

Stadium	n	n	mit positiven Knoten
IIIa	11	5	45%
IIIb	10	6	60%
IIIc	98	81	83%
Gesamt	119	92	77%

In der überwiegenden Mehrzahl waren eine bis zwei Lymphknotengruppen von Karzinomabsiedelungen betroffen. Ein ausgedehnter metastatischer Befall mit 7 oder 8 positiven Drüsengruppen kam jedoch auch vor.

Mit der Zahl der metastatisch befallenen Lymphknoten nehmen auch die Tumorabsiedelungen in ihnen an Größe zu. Dies kann auch als ein weiterer Beweis für die positive Korrelation zwischen dem Grad der Tumorausbreitung und der absoluten Tumormasse gewertet werden.

Die *topographische* Verteilung der metastatisch befallenen Lymphknoten des kleinen Beckens zeigte keine Regelhaftigkeit (Abb. 1). Die Metastasen in den Lymphknoten beider Beckenhälften wurden etwa gleich häufig aufgefunden. Am häufigsten waren jeweils die externen iliacalen Lymphknoten metastatisch befallen [10]. Allerdings beobachteten WU et al. [17] eine besondere Beziehung zwischen dem Primärsitz des Ovarialkarzinoms und der Lateralität der Lymphknotenmetastasen: So konnten sie feststellen, daß die Metastasenfrequenz in den Lymphknoten mit 71% bei Bilateralität des Ovarialkarzinoms am höchsten ist. Bei Unilateralität wurde gefunden, daß der linksseitige karzinomatöse Ovarialbefall mit 45%, also um vieles häufiger zu Lymphknotenmetastasen führt, als wenn nur das rechte Ovar karzinomatös befallen war, in welchem Fall nur 8% der Lymphknoten betroffen waren (Tabelle 6). Diese Befunde können am eigenen Material allerdings nicht wirklich bestätigt werden, wenn auch bei alleinigem linksseitigen Befall (n=30) Lymphknotenmetastasen in 50% und bei rechtsseitigem Befall (n=36) noduläre Absiedelungen in 39% gefunden werden.

Der weitere lymphatische Abfluß sowohl aus dem Zwerchfell als auch aus dem diaphragmalen Pleuraabschnitten erfolgt zum einen Teil in die mediastinalen Lymphknoten und danach in die supraclaviculären und präskalenischen Lymphknoten. Zum anderen führt der Abstrom direkt in die Cisterna chyli bzw. in den Ductus thoracicus und in den Subclavia-Venenwinkel [16]. Damit ist die Möglichkeit der Verschleppung der Tumorzellen in den Blutkreislauf gegeben. Der Nachweis von Metastasen in die präskalenischen Lymphknoten ist ein wichtiger Indikator für die Generalisierung dieser Tumorkrankheit und erlaubt zusammen mit der Feststellung der intraabdominalen Tumormasse eine gute Beurteilung des Schweregrades der Erkrankung [5,7,10,12]. Dies kann sehr gut an dem markanten Anstieg der Metastasenfrequenz in den präskalenischen Lymphknoten im Stadium IV gegenüber dem Stadium III abgelesen werden (Tabelle 7).

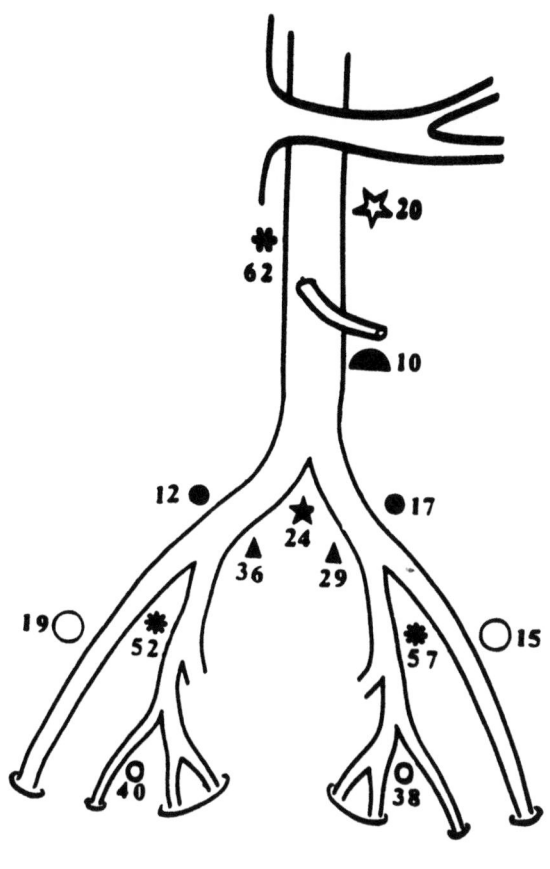

Abb. 1: *Topographische* Verteilung der metastatisch befallenen Lymphknoten des kleinen Beckens

Tabelle 6: Primärsitz der Ovarialkarzinome und Frequenz der pelvinen Lymphknotenmetastasen [nach 17]

Primärsitz	n	positive Knoten				
		links	rechts	bilateral	gesamt	(%)
linkes Ovar	38	5	5	7	17	(45)
rechtes Ovar	35	0	2	0	2	(8)
bilateral	42	3	5	22	30	(71)
Gesamt	105	8	12	29	49	(47)

Tabelle 7: Metastatischer Befall der Scalenuslymphknoten bei 37 Patienten mit Ovarialkarzinom

Stadium	n	Scalenuslymphknoten positiv	
I	3	0	(0)
II	2	0	(0)
III	25	3	(12%)
IV	7	4	(57%)
Gesamt	37	7	(21%)

Zusammenfassung

Das Ovarialkarzinom breitet sich einerseits auf transabdominellem Wege aus und erreicht verhältnismäßig rasch den Oberbauch, wobei die Möglichkeit einer Tumorentstehung de novo auf der Peritonealoberfläche mit sekundärer Implantationsmetastasierung offen bleibt. Andererseits setzt das Ovarialkarzinom über die lymphatischen Gefäßbahnen Metastasen in die pelvinen und paraaortalen Lymphknoten. Das heißt, daß sich das Ovarialkarzinom fast parallel in zwei Bereichen, nämlich intraabdominell und retroperitoneal, ausbreitet.

Literatur

1. August C.Z., Murad T.M., Newton M.: Multiple focal extraovarian serous carcinoma. Int. J. Gynecol. Pathol. 4: 11-23, 1985
2. Averette H.E., Lovecchio J.L., Townsend P.A.: Retroperitoneal lymphatic involvement by ovarian carcinoma. In: Cancer Campaign Carcinoma of the ovary. Fischer, Stuttgart 7: 101, 1983
3. Barber H.R.K.: Spread and treatment of advanced ovarian cancer. Bailliére's Clin. Obstet. Gynecol. 3: 23-29, 1989
4. Buchsbaum H.J., Brady M.F., Delgado G. et al.: Surgical staging of carcinoma of the ovaries. Surg. Gynecol. Obstet. 169: 226-235, 1989
5. Burghardt E., Lahousen M., Stettner H.: Die operative Behandlung des Ovarialkarzinoms. Geburtsh. Frauenheilk. 50: 670-677, 1990
6. Burghardt E., Girardi F., Lahousen M., Tamussino K., Stettner H.: Patterns of pelvic and paraaortic lymph node involvement in ovarian cancer. Gynecol. Oncol. 40: 103-106, 1991
7. Burke T.W., Heller P.B., Hoskins W.J.: Evaluation of the scalene lymph nodes in primary and recurrent cervical carcinoma. Gynecol. Oncol. 28: 312-317, 1987
8. Chen S.S., Lee L.: Incidence of para-aortic and pelvic lymph node metastases in epithelial carcinoma of the ovary. Gynecol. Oncol. 16: 95-100, 1983
9. Fuks Z.: Patterns of spread of ovarian carcinoma: relation to therapeutic strategies. In Newman C.E., Ford C., Jordan J.H. (eds) Ovarian Cancer: 39-51, 1989
10. Pickel H., Lahousen M., Stettner H., Girardi F.: The spread of ovarian cancer. Bailliére's Clin. Obstet. Gynecol. 3: 3-13, 1989
11. Plentl A.A., Friedman E.A.: Lymphatic system of the female genitalia in Major Problems. In: Obstetrics and Gynecology (eds. E.A. Friedman) Philadelphia, Saunders: 173, 1973
12. Posawetz W., Jakse R., Petru E., Pickel H., Heydarfadai M.: Die Skalenusbiopsie in der Diagnostik von Ovarial- und Uteruskarzinomen. HNO: 367-369, 1990
13. Rose P.G., Piver M.S., Tsukada Y., Lau T.: Metastatic patterns in histologic variants of ovarian cancer. Cancer 64: 1508-1513, 1989
14. Sevin B.U.: Intraoperative staging in ovarian cancer. Bailliére's Clin. Obstet. Gynecol. 3: 13-21, 1989
15. Tobacman J.A., Tucker M.A., Kase R.: Intraabdominal carcinomatosis after prophylactic oophorectomy in ovarian-cancer-prone families. Lancet ii: 795-798, 1982
16. Williams P.L., Warwick R.: Gray's Anatomy. Edinburgh Churchill: 798, 1980
17. Wu P.C.H., Lang J.H., Huang R.L., Qu J.Y.: Lymph node metastases and retroperitoneal lymphadnecetomy in ovarian cancer. Bailliére's Clin. Obstet. Gynaecol. 3: 143-155, 1989

Follow-up unter Chemotherapie: Welche Bedeutung haben die Tumormarker für die Prognoseeinschätzung?

R. Kreienberg

Zweifelsohne stellt das Ovarialkarzinom das Problemkarzinom auch im Bereich der Nachsorge dar. Jährlich erkranken ca. 15 von 100.000 Frauen an einer malignen Neubildung des Ovars. Die Inzidenz dieses Organmalignoms scheint ansteigend zu sein. Charakteristische Symptome, die frühzeitig auf eine maligne Erkrankung des Ovars hinweisen würden, fehlen, sodaß mehr als zwei Drittel aller Patientinnen erst in fortgeschrittenen Tumorstadien der Primärbehandlung zugeführt werden.

Die Prognose der Erkrankung wird entscheidend vom Tumorstadium bei der Primärtherapie beeinflußt. Weitere Prognosekriterien sind daneben bekanntermaßen der Allgemeinzustand, das Alter der Patientin, der histologische Typ und der Differenzierungsgrad der Tumorzellen sowie die nach der Primärtherapie verbliebene Resttumormasse. Zusätzlich zu diesen genannten Faktoren ist es von besonderem Interesse, ob bestimmte Laborparameter, präoperativ, postoperativ oder im weiteren Verlauf bestimmt, in der Lage sind, prognostische Informationen zu liefern, die die aktuell vorhandene Tumormasse, den jeweiligen Therapieerfolg und auch die Langzeitprognose voraussagen lassen.

Im Folgenden soll Stellung genommen werden, welche Bedeutung Tumormarker für die Prognoseeinschätzung beim Ovarialkarzinom haben.

Tumormarker im Rahmen der Primärtherapie

Der klinisch geeigneteste Tumormarker beim Ovarialkarzinom schien anfangs das karzinoembryonale Antigen zu sein. Deutliche Fortschritte in der Markeranwendung beim Ovarialkarzinom haben sich erst durch die Einführung des Cancer Antigen 125 (CA 125) ergeben. Durch diesen Marker werden überwiegend serös-papilläre und undifferenzierte Adenokarzinome des Ovars nachgewiesen [4,5]. Es konnte gezeigt werden, daß die Sensitivität von CA 125-Bestimmungen im Serum präoperativ in Abhängigkeit vom Stadium der Tumoren zwischen 43 und 83% liegt und stadienabhängig ansteigt [3,6].

Bei einem oberen Grenzwert von 65 U/ml findet sich eine Spezifität für gesunde Kontrollpersonen von 99%, für Patientinnen mit benignen Adnexprozessen von 92% und für Patientinnen mit Enzündungen von 83% [3,6]. Der Anteil der richtig-positiven prätherapeutischen Befunde sind neben dem Stadium der Tumorerkrankung auch von dem histologischen Tumortyp abhängig. 90% der undifferenzierten Ovarialkarzinome, 80% der serös-papillären Karzinome des Ovars, 62% der endometrioiden und 40% der muzinösen Karzinome weisen richtig-positive Serumkonzentrationen dieses Markers auf.

Die Höhe der präoperativ gemessenen Serumspiegel von CA 125 korrelieren direkt mit der vor der Operation vorhandenen Tumormasse. In gleicher Weise korrelieren die postoperativ gemessenen Serumkonzentrationen von CA 125 mit dem verbliebenen Tumorrest. Die zu diesem Zeitpunkt gemessenen Serumkonzentrationen dieses Markers stellen somit keinen eigenständigen Prognoseparameter dar, sondern sind sowohl prä- als auch postoperativ von der tatsächlich vorhandenen Tumormasse und damit von den beiden wesentlichen prognostischen Parameter wie Tumorstadium und postoperativ verbliebenen Tumorrest abhängig.

Trotzdem ist der präoperativ gemessene CA 125-Serumspiegel ein indirektes Maß für die vor der Operation vorhandene tatsächliche Tumormasse, die durch die Stadieneinteilung nach FIGO ja nur ungenügend beschrieben wird.

Die Differenz zwischen den prä- und postoperativ gemessenen Serumspiegeln dieses Markers repräsentiert die durch die Operation erreichte Tumorreduktion.

Die Höhe des postoperativ gemessenen Serumspiegels von CA 125 ist als Ausgangspunkt für die Beurteilung der Effektivität der sich an die Operation anschließenden, zur Beseitigung des Resttumors dringend notwendigen Chemotherapie, von besonderer Bedeutung.

Tumormarker in der Verlaufskontrolle

Die CA 125-Serumkonzentrationen im weiteren Krankheitsverlauf kontrolliert, geben relativ exakt die jeweils vorhandene Tumoraktivität wieder. Abbildung 1 zeigt in Einzelverläufen, daß präoperativ über den Grenzwert von 65 U/ml erhöhte CA 125-Werte nach suffizienter Primärtherapie sich normalisieren und bei Rezidivfreiheit im Normbereich verbleiben. Patientinnen mit nur geringer Tumorreduktion, bei denen überwiegend Probelaparatomien durchge-

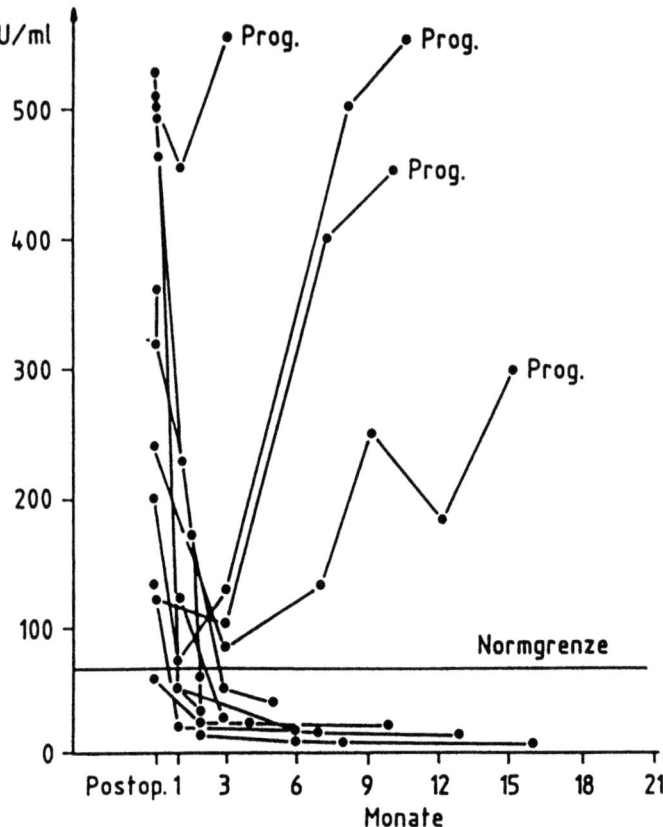

Abb. 1: Verläufe individueller CA 125-Serumspiegel bei Patientinnen mit Ovarialkarzinomen präoperativ, postoperativ (postop.), bei Rezidivfreiheit und bei Progredienz (Prog.), Überwachungsbereich präoperativ und postoperativ in Monaten

führt werden konnten, weisen nur kurzzeitige Serumkonzentrationserniedrigungen dieses Markers auf. Der Wiederanstieg der CA 125-Werte zeigt die Progredienz des jeweiligen Tumormarkers an. Gleiches läßt sich in einer Sammelstatistik der GTMG zeigen [1,3,6]. Bei erfolgreicher Primärbehandlung fanden sich nur bei 1% der rezidivfreien Frauen (NED=no evidence for diseases) erhöhte Serumkonzentrationen. Patientinnen mit einem rezidivierten oder progredienten Ovarialkarzinom wiesen dagegen in 74 bsw. 79% der Fälle CA 125-Werte von über 65 U/ml auf.

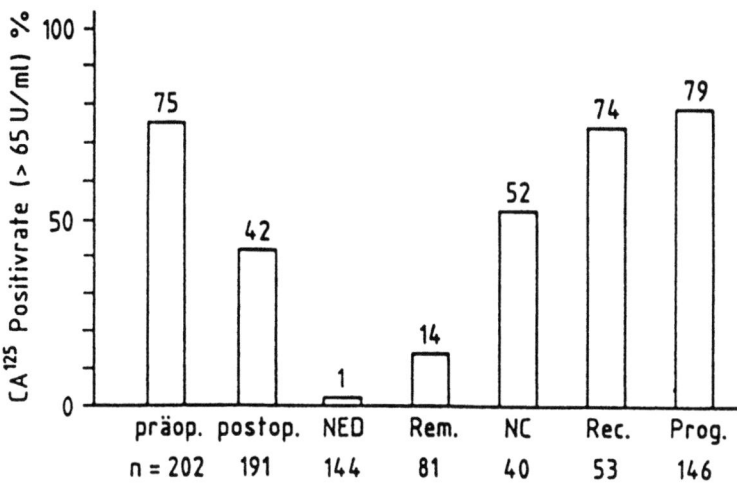

Abb. 2: Verlaufsuntersuchungen bei Patientinnen mit Ovarialkarzinomen (NED=No evidence for disease; Rem.=Remmission, NC=No change, Rec.=Rezidiv, Prog.=Progression) [nach GTMG 9]

Damit wird deutlich, daß sich mit Hilfe konsekutiver Serumbestimmungen von CA 125 der Erfolg der Chemotherapie voraussagen läßt und die Früherkennung des Rezidivs bzw. einer Progredienz des Tumorwachstums möglich ist.

Besonders interessant sind in diesem Zusammenhang Untersuchungen, die überprüft haben, welche prognostische Information in der Geschwindigkeit des Abfalls des CA 125-Serumspiegels unter Chemotherapie liegt. Van der Burg et al. [8], Hawkins et al. [2] und Mogensen et al. [7] konnten zeigen, daß die Halbierung der CA 125-Serumkonzentrationen unter einer Chemotherapie in einem Zeitraum von weniger als 20 Tagen zu einer Steigerung der kompletten Remissionsraten und zu einer signifikanten Verlängerung der Überlebenszeit führt.

Damit scheint der Steilheit des Abfalls der CA 125-Serumkonzentration unter Chemotherapie eine eigenständige prognostische Bedeutung zuzukommen. Dies muß jedoch an größeren Patientinnenkollektiven noch überprüft werden.

Tabelle 1: CA 125 beim Ovarialkarzinom: Serumspiegel uns Second-look-Befunde (Daten der Arbeitsgruppen UFK Würzburg, Heidelberg und Mainz) (Anzahl (n) Patienten) [nach 6]

Präoperativ (vor SL-Op)		Anzahl Pat. total	Intraoperativer Befund bei SL-Op				
CA 125 [b]	Klinisch		Tumor makroskop.			Tumor mikroskop.[a]	
			>2cm	≤2cm	Tu-frei	positiv	negativ
Negativ	Tu-negativ	40	-	4	36	8	28
Positiv	Tu-negativ	3	1	1	1	1	0
Negativ	Tu-positiv	4	2	2	-	-	-
Positiv	Tu-positiv	7	3	4	-	-	-
Total mit SL-Op		54	6	11	37	9	28

a Nur für makroskopisch Tu-freie Patienten, makroskopischer Rest-Tu wurde jeweils auch histologisch bestätigt
b Grenzwert 65 U/ml (Streuungsbereich negativer Patienten <5-32, positiver 74-419)

Tumormarker und Second-look-Befunde

Für den Kliniker besonders wichtig ist die Frage, inwieweit sich mit Hilfe der CA 125-Serumbestimmung die bei der Second-look-Operation erhobenen klinischen und histologischen Befunde voraussagen lassen. Tabelle 1 zeigt, daß Patientinnen mit CA 125-Werten über 65 U/ml trotz klinisch negativer Befunderhebung vor der Second-look-Operation (unter Einschluß aller radiologischen Methoden) in allen Fällen makroskopische oder mikroskopische Tumorreste im Abdomen aufweisen.

Bei Patientinnen mit CA 125-Serumkonzentrationen im Normbereich (unter 65 U/ml) findet sich dagegen in 70% der Fälle (28/40) weder makroskopisch noch mikroskopisch bei der Second-look-Operation ein Tumorrest. Bei Patientinnen mit klinisch-negativen Tumorbefund bei erhöhten CA 125 Serumkonzentrationen über 65 U/ml läßt sich somit die reine Inspektions-Secondlook-Laparatomie vermeiden. Bei Patientinnen mit klinisch-negativem Tumorbefund und normalen CA 125-Serumkonzentrationen kann nur in zwei Drittel der Fälle von einer Tumorfreiheit ausgegangen werden.

Zusammenfassung

Die heute bekannten Tumormarker sind alle Stoffwechsel- oder Syntheseprodukte, die direkt aus der Tumorzelle stammen und an das Serum weitergegeben werden. Diese Marker stellen keine eigenständigen Prognoseparameter dar, sondern reflektieren die jeweils vorhandene Tumormasse. Prognostische Bedeutung ergibt sich dadurch, daß sich aus ihren Veränderungen unter Therapie deren Erfolg und damit die Prognose der Erkrankung ablesen läßt. Präoperative CA 125-Spiegel repräsentieren das Tumorstadium, postoperative Serumspiegel korrelieren mit der Radikalität der Operation und dem nach der Operation verbliebenen Tumorrest. Der weitere Abfall der CA 125-Serumspiegel unter Chemotherapie beweist den Effekt dieser therapeutischen Maßnahme.

Inwieweit sich aus der Geschwindigkeit des Abfalls der CA 125-Serumkonzentrationen unter Chemotherapie der Anteil der Remissionen und das Überleben prognostizieren läßt, ist eine überaus interessante Fragestellung, die erst nach weiteren Untersuchungen endgültig beantwortet werden kann. Serumkonzentrationen von CA 125 über 65 U/ml deuten in 100% der Fälle auf Tumorrest im Abdomen hin und machen die reine Second-look-Laparatomie überflüssig. Bei Patientinnen mit CA 125-Serumkonzentrationen unter 65 U/ml ist die Voraussage der Tumorfreiheit nur in 70% der Fälle korrekt. Im Rahmen der Nachsorge zeigen wiederansteigende Tumormarker-Serumkonzentrationen in über 80% der Fälle frühzeitig das Rezidiv bzw. die Progredienz des Tumorwachstums an.

Sicher ist, daß die Tumormarker-Serumkonzentrationen zum Zeitpunkt der Metastasierung gemessen, zur Prognosebeurteilung des weiteren Krankheitsverlaufes als Effektivitätsbeurteilung von Second- bzw. Third-line-Therapien herangezogen werden können.

Literatur

1. Caffier H., Crombach G., Kaufmann M., Kreienberg R.: CA 125 im Serum. Second-look-Befunde und Langzeitprognosen des Ovarialkarzinoms. 4. Hamburger Symposium über Tumormarker. Greten H., Klapdor R. (Hrsg.) Thieme, Stuttgart New York: 393, 1987
2. Hawkins R.E., Roberts K., Wiltshaw E., Mundy J., Fryatt I.J., Mc Cready V.R.: The prognostic significance of the halflife of serum CA 125 in patients responding to chemotherapy for epithelial ovarian carcinoma. Brit. J. Obstr. Gynaecol. 96: 1395-1399, 1989

3. Kaesemann H., Caffier H., Hoffmann F.J., Crombach S., Würz H., Kreienberg R., Möbus V., Schmidt-Rhode P., Sturm G.: Monoklonale Antikörper in Diagnostik und Verlaufskontrolle des Ovarialkarzinoms. CA 125 als Tumormarker. Eine kooperative Studie der Gynäkologischen Tumormarkergruppe (GTMG). Klin. Wochenschr. 64: 781, 1986
4. Kreienberg R.: Allgemeine und spezifische Laborparameter im Rahmen der Tumornachsorge bei gynäkologischen Malignomen und bei Mammakarzinomen. Gynäkologe 22: 55-62, 1989
5. Kreienberg R., Möbus V.: Tumormarker in der Gynäkologie (Tumor markers in breast cancer and gynecological tumors). Lab. med. 16: 21-26, 1992
6. Möbus V., Kreienberg R., Crombach G., Würz H., Caffier H., Kaesemann H., Hoffmann F.J., Schmidt-Rhode P., Sturm G., Kaufmann M.: Evaluation of CA 125 as a prognostic and predictive factor in ovarian cancer. Symposiumband 4th. Intern. Conference of human tumor markers. J. Tumor Marker Oncol. 3.1: 251-258, 1988
7. Mogensen O., Mogensen B., Jakobsen A.: Predictive value of CA 125 during early chemotherapy of advanced ovarian cancer. Gynecol. Oncol. 37: 44-46, 1990
8. Van der Burg M.E.L., Lames F.B., Van Putten W.L.J., Stoter G.: Ovarian cancer: The prognostic value of the serum half-life of CA 125 during induction chemotherapy. Gynecol. Oncol. 30: 307-312, 1988

Evaluation of the Serum Markers CA 125, CA 15.3 and CA M29 in Monitoring Ovarian Cancer

M.E.L. van der Burg[1], G. Bon[2], R. Oosterom[1], A. Verstraeten[2], G. van Kamp[2], C. Yedema[2], L. Rozendaal[2], J. Vermorken[2], P. Kenemans[2]

Introduction

In ovarian cancer, known as the »hidden« tumor, difficulties are encountered in the evaluation of the effectiveness of therapy and in diagnosing progressive or recurrent disease at an early stage. Given the tumor's distinctive pattern of spread over serosal surfaces, advanced ovarian cancer is frequently associated with multiple small metastatic tumor deposits which stud the parietal and visceral peritoneum [7]. Small residual tumor nodules cannot be detected by the most careful gynecological or general physical examination nor by the most sophisticated methods like computerized tomography [2]. Chemotherapy therefore may be given for several months without knowing whether the residual tumor is regressing or progressing. In this setting a tumor marker, which accurately reflects tumor burden, would improve the management of ovarian cancer by preventing ineffective treatment mostly accompanied by severe toxicity.

The serum tumor marker CA 125, found to be elevated in 82% of the patients with epithelial ovarian cancer, is a reliable tumor marker to diagnose progression in an early stage [1]. However, 30% of the patients have normal serum CA 125 levels at the diagnosis of clinical progression [3]. The serum markers CA 15.3 and CA M29, both detecting mucinic antigens, were found to be increased in respectively 71% and 60% of the ovarian cancer patients [6,10]. By combining the measurement of CA 125 with CA 15.3 and CA M29 the (early) detection of progressive disease might be improved.

In this study we investigated the accuracy of the concomitant measurement of the serum markers CA 125, CA 15.3 and CA M29 in diagnosing progressive or recurrent disease at an early stage.

---

1 Rotterdam Cancer Institute; Daniel den Hoed Kliniek, Rotterdam
2 Free University Hospital Amsterdam, Amsterdam

Patients and Methods

A total of hundred-thirteen patients were entered in the study. All patients were treated according to protocols with combination chemotherapy. Tumor response was monitored according to protocols by means of gynecological and general physical examination, complete blood counts and 12 channel biochemical screen performed prior to every chemotherapy cycle and at every follow-up visit. CT-scan and chest film were performed after every third chemotherapy cycle and once a year during follow up. Patient records were evaluated separately from the marker values. Progression was defined according to the WHO response criteria [9].

Serum samples for marker determinations were taken prior to chemotherapy cycles and at follow-up visits, stored at -70°C and measured en bloc at the end of the study period. The interval between serum sampling ranged from 3 weeks to 6 months pending the interval between the chemotherapy cycles (3-5 weeks) and control visits (2-6 months). All serum assays were performed according to the manufacturer's instructions. The upper limit of normal used for CA 125, CA 15.3 (both RIA, Centocor) and CA M29 (EIA, Genetic Systems) were 35 U/ml, 30 U/ml and 15 U/ml, respectively.

Results

Hundred-thirteen patients were evaluable. During a minimum-follow-up of 5 years, 77 patients developed progressive disease. The patient characteristics of these patients were the following: stage according to FIGO, stage I 7 patients, stage II 13 patients, stage III 34 patients and stage IV disease 23 patients. Histological types included: 26 serous, 9 endometrioid, 7 mucinous, 6 clear-cell, 29 undifferentiated adenocarcinomas. Histological grade was: grade 1 in 3 patients, grade 2 in 15 patients, grade 3 in 39 patients and unknown in 20 patients.

At the time of clinical diagnosis of progression CA 125 was increased in 70% of the patients, CA 15.3 in 55%, CA M29 in 60% and an increase of one of the three markers was found in 79% (fig. 1). An increase of the marker before clinical evidence of progression was found for CA 125 in 61%, for CA 15.3 in 43% and for CA M29 in 48% of the patients and for one of the 3 markers in 70% of the patients. In the patients with an increased CA 125 6% had an increase of CA 15.3 and / or CA M29 before the rise of CA 125. Moreover 10% of the patients with a normal CA 125 at progression had an increased CA 15.3

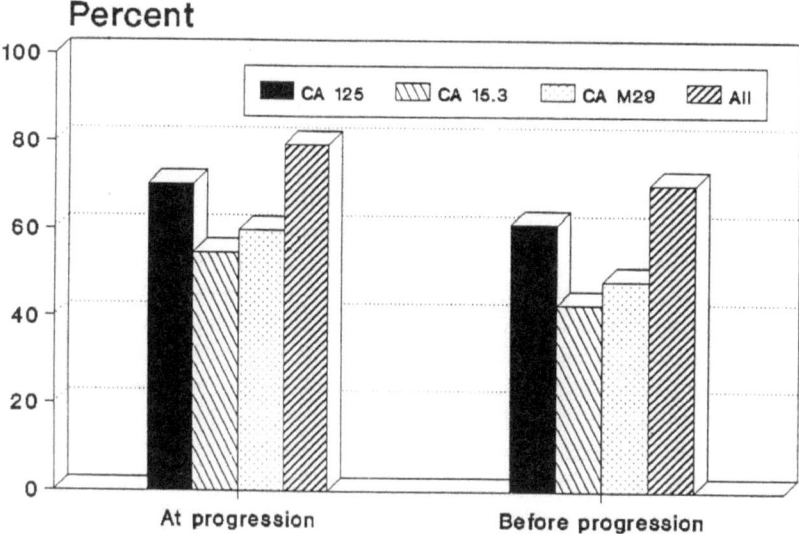

Fig. 1: Marker increase and progression

and / or CA M29. The median lead-time for all 3 markers was about 4.5 months with a range of 1 to 25 months. No significant difference in lead-time has been observed between the 3 markers. Neither FIGO stage nor histological subtype or grade did significantly influence the increase for the different markers.

Thirty-six patients had no evidence of disease after a median follow-up of 7 years, range 5 to 9 years. During this period a total of 180 serum samples have been evaluated. A false positive increased serum marker was found for CA 125, CA 15.3 and CA M29 in 1,7%, 6,7% and 6,7% respectively. An increase of one of the 3 markers was observed in 14,4%.

Discussion

Early diagnosis of progressive or recurrent disease in ovarian cancer is hampered by the usually prolonged symptomless period of tumor growth [7]. Consequently quite a number of patients are treated during a shorter or longer period of time with an ineffective toxic therapy. CA 125 proved to be an effective marker in monitoring ovarian cancer [1,3]. However, 30% of the patients with progressive disease have a normal CA 125 value. The present study was initiated to define the complementary use of the markers CA 15.3 and CA M29 to the clinical established marker CA 125.

From the 3 markers CA 125 is still the most reliable marker to detect progression in an early stage. An increase of CA 125 before clinical progression was observed in 61% of the patients in regard to 43% and 48% for CA 15.3 and CA M29, respectively (fig. 1). The lead-time from serum increase to progression was median 4.5 months and was the same for the 3 markers. With the additional measurement of the markers CA 15.3 and CA M29 to CA 125, it was possible to detect progression earlier in 16% of the patients. The false positive rate in the 36 patients with no evidence of disease during a median follow-up of 7 years was for CA 125 1,7% and for CA 15.3 and CA M29 6,7% respectively. An increase of one of the 3 markers was observed in 14.4%. However, these increases were marginal and significantly lower than in patients with progressive disease. More or less the same results have been observed by the combination of CA 125 with MCA, CA 19.9, LSA, NB/70K and PIIINP [4,5,8].

In conclusion: Serum CA 125 proved to be the most useful marker in the early detection of progressive disease in ovarian cancer. The concomitant measurement of CA 15.3 and CA M29 further increases the accuracy of early detection of progression in an additional 16% of patients.

References

1. Bast R.C., Klug T.L., John E.S. et al.: A radioimmunoassay using a monoclonal antibody to monitor the course of epithelial ovarian cancer. N. Engl. J. Med. 309: 883-887, 1983
2. Brenner D.E., Shaff M.I., Jones H.W. et al.: Abdominopelvic computed tomography: evaluation in patients undergoing second-look laparotomy for ovarian carcinoma. Obstet. Gynecol. 65: 715-719, 1985
3. Van der Burg M.E.L., Lammes F.B., Verwey J.: The role of CA 125 in the early detection of progressive disease in ovarian cancer. An. Oncol. 1: 301-302, 1990
4. Koelbl H., Schieder K., Neunteufel W. et al.: A Comparative study of mucin-like carcinoma-associated antigen (MCA), CA 125, CA 19.9 and CEA in patients with ovarian cancer. Neoplasma 36: 473-478, 1989
5. Petru E., Sevin B.U., Averette H.E. et al.: Comparison of three tumor markers CA 125, lipid associated sialic acid (SLA) and NB/70K in monitoring ovarian cancer. Gynecol. Oncol. 38: 181-186, 1990

6. Scambia G., Benedetti Panici P., Baiocchi G. et al.: CA 15.3 as a tumor marker in gynecological malignancies. Gynecol. Oncol. 30: 265-273, 1988
7. Smith L.H., Ol R.H.: Detection of malignant ovarian neoplasms: a review of the literature. Detection of the patient at risk ; clinical, radiological and cytological detection. Obstet. Gynecol. Survey. 39: 323-328, 1984
8. Tomas C., Penttinen J., Risteli L. et al.: Simultaneous evaluation of epithelial cell function by CA 125 and stromal cell activity by aminoterminal propeptide of type III procollagen (PIIINP) in ovarian carcinoma. An. Med. 22: 115-121, 1990
9. WHO Handbook for Reporting results of cancer treatment. Geneva WHO, WHO Offset Publication no 48, 1979
10. Yedema K.A., Kenemans P., Wobbes T. et al.: Carcinoma associated mucin serum markers CA M26 and CA M29: Efficacy in detecting and monitoring patients with cancer of the breast, colon, ovary, endometrium and cervix. Int. J. Cancer 47: 170-179, 1991

Rezeptorstatus und Überlebenszeit beim Ovarialkarzinom

M. Krohn, G. Trams

Es ist bekannt, daß Ovarialkarzinome Östrogen- und Progesteronrezeptoren enthalten können. Ungeklärt ist, ob in Bezug auf die Prognose, die Behandlungsstrategie und eine evtl. hormonelle Substitution der Rezeptorstatus relevant ist.

Beim gegenwärtigen Wissensstand kann es nicht darum gehen, endgültige Antworten auf die skizzierten Fragen zu geben. Es kann nur darum gehen, durch Korrelation des Rezeptorstatus mit klinischen Daten einen partiellen Beitrag zur Eingrenzung der Problemstellungen zu leisten. Dieses war unser Anspruch an die Auswertung von 159 Rezeptoranalysen von Ovarialkarzinomen.

Die Rezeptorbefunde korrelierten wir mit dem Alter der Patientinnen, der Histologie, dem Tumorstadium, der postoperativen Resttumorgröße und der Überlebenszeit. Die Rezeptorbestimmung erfolgte nach der DCC-Methode, der Grenzwert lag bei 20 fmol pro mg Cytosolprotein.

Häufigkeitsverteilung

In 62% war entweder der Östrogen- oder der Progesteronrezeptor positiv. 27% der Rezeptorproben waren sowohl östrogen- als auch progesteronrezeptorpositiv. Es waren mehr Karzinome progesteronrezeptorpositiv als östrogenrezeptorpositiv (50% vs. 38%) (Abb. 1).

Menopausenstatus

58% der prämenopausalen Patientinnen waren rezeptorpositiv, im Vergleich zu 64% der postmenopausalen Patientinnen. Der Unterschied ist nicht signifikant. Ähnliche Ergebnisse finden sich in der Literatur [1,8,9,12,17,18].

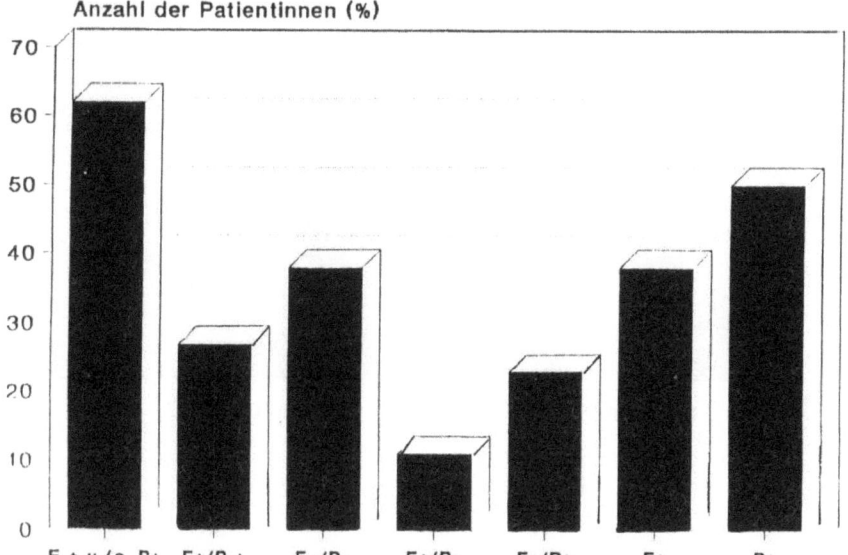

Abb. 1: Rezeptorverteilung (n=159)

Histologie und Rezeptorstatus

Das unklassifizierbare und das adenopapilläre Karzinom waren die häufigsten histologischen Diagnosen. Eine Beziehung zwischen Histologie und Rezeptorstatus konnten wir an unserem Untersuchungsmaterial nicht beobachten. In der Literatur finden sich einige wenige Arbeiten, die eine Korrelation postulieren für kleine Subgruppen [6,7,18,19].

Tumorstadium und Rezeptorstatus

Ca. 1/3 der Patientinnen wurde im Stadium I und II operiert, 2/3 im Stadium III und IV. Im Stadium I und II waren 85% rezeptorpositiv. Im Stadium III und IV waren es 57% (Abb. 2). Diese Zahlen spiegeln eine Tendenz zur höheren Rezeptorpositivität in den Frühstadien. Auch Spona [16] fand ein gehäuftes Vorkommen von Östrogen- und Progesteronrezeptoren in den Stadien I und II, mehrheitlich wird dieses Ergebnis jedoch nicht bestätigt.

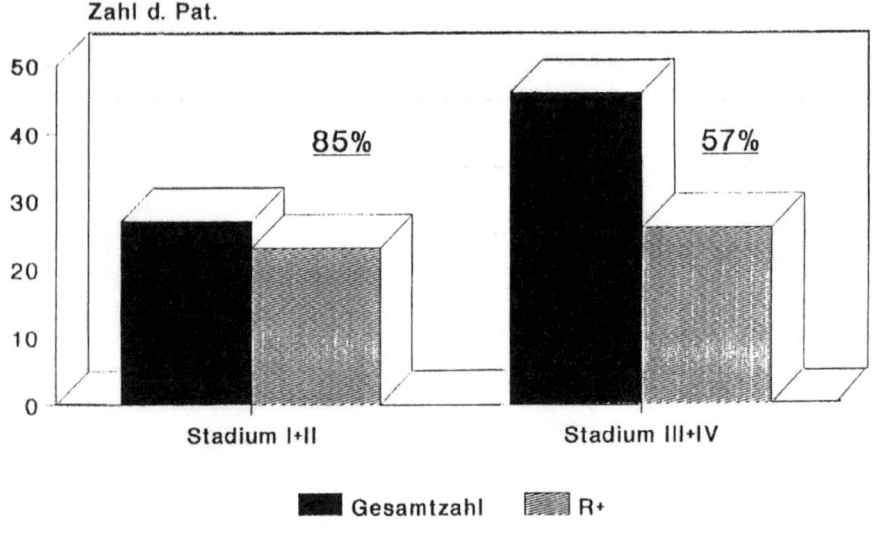

Abb. 2: FIGO-Stadien und Rezeptorstatus E+ u./o. P+ (n=73)

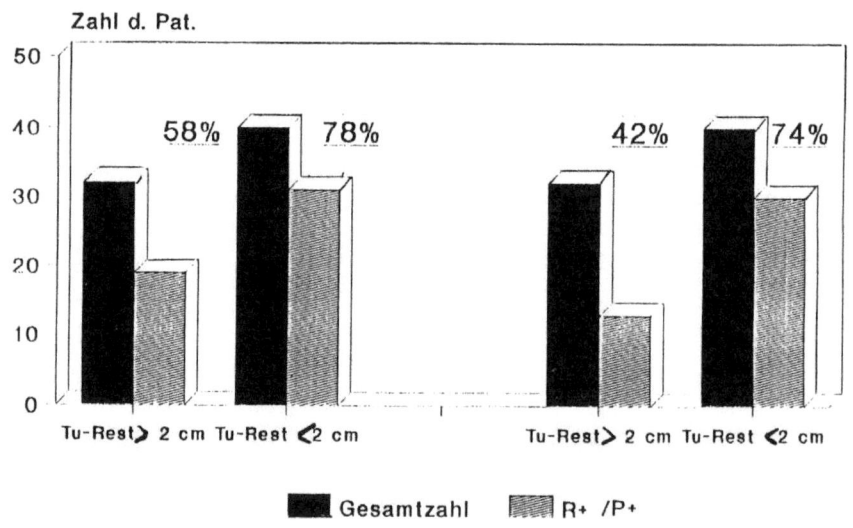

Abb. 3: Tumorrest und Rezeptorstatus E+ u./o. P+ (n=72)

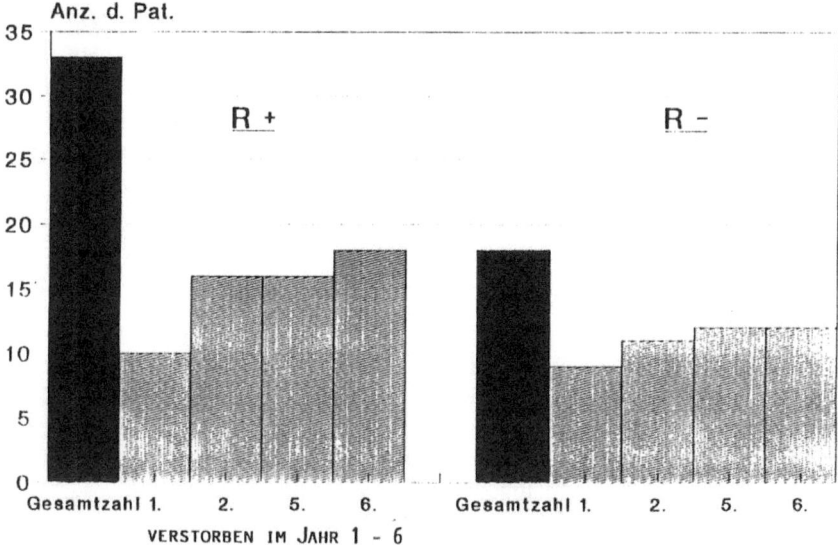

Abb. 4: Rezeptorstatus und Überleben (n=51)

Tumorrest und Rezeptorstatus

Bei einer Resttumorgröße über 2 cm lag in 58% ein positiver Rezeptorstatus vor, bei einer Resttumorgröße unter 2 cm in 78% (Abb. 3, linke Bildhälfte). Der Unterschied ist nicht signifikant. Der Unterschied ausschließlich in Bezug auf den Östrogenrezeptor ist ebenfalls nicht signifikant. Signifikant war allerdings die Differenz hinsichtlich des Progesteronrezeptorstatus (Abb. 3, rechte Bildhälfte): Ovarialkarzinome, die unter 2 cm Resttumor operiert werden konnten, enthielten signifikant häufiger Progesteronrezeptoren mit einem höheren Progesteronrezeptorgehalt (42% vs. 74%; $p = 0{,}0009$ — errechnet mit dem t-Test für unabhängige Stichproben bei ungleicher Varianz).

Überlebenszeit

Der Median der Nachbeobachtungszeit betrug 4,3 Jahre, das Minimum lag bei 1 Jahr, das Maximum betrug 11 Jahre. 30 Patientinnen sind verstorben, 18 waren rezeptorpositiv, 12 negativ, der Unterschied ist nicht signifikant. Von den 21 lebenden Patientinnen sind 15 rezeptorpositiv, 6 negativ. Untersucht man die Überlebenszeiten nach 1,2,5 und 6 Jahren, ergeben sich keine signifikanten Unterschiede hinsichtlich des Rezeptorstatus. Im 1. Jahr waren 10 von 33 rezeptorpositiven Patientinnen verstorben (30%) und 9 von 18 rezeptornegativen (50%). Die leichten Unterschiede sind bereits nach 2 Jahren aufgehoben (50% vs. 60%) (Abb. 4). Zu ähnlichen Ergebnissen gelangen zahlreiche andere Autoren [1,4,9,10,11,12,13,18].

Vereinzelt konnten in kleinen Untergruppen Tendenzen, keine Signifikanzen zu günstigeren Überlebenszeiten errechnet werden, z.t. mit sich widersprechenden Ergebnissen [2,3,5,6,14,15,19].

Ob die Bestimmung von Rezeptoren bei Ovarialkarzinomen klinisch verwertbare Informationen bietet, ist ungewiß. Sich widersprechende Literaturergebnisse können Ausdruck der tatsächlich fehlenden Relevanz sein, können aber auch im Zusammenhang mit kleinen Fallzahlen stehen. Unsere Untersuchung ist einerseits nur eine quantitative Ergänzung bisher vorliegender Studien. Andererseits kann besser gesichertes Wissen auch nur empirisch gewonnen werden — über die Kumulation zahlreicher ähnlicher Untersuchungen.

Zu den auffälligsten Beobachtungen der vorgetragenen Auswertung gehören:

1. Keine Beziehung Rezeptorstatus/Menopausenstatus
2. Keine Beziehung Rezeptorstatus/Histologie
3. Tendenz zu höherem Rezeptorvorkommen im Stadium I und II
4. Resttumorgröße unter 2 cm bei signifikant höherem Progesteronrezeptorgehalt
5. Keine bessere Überlebenszeit bei rezeptorpositivem Tumor

Literatur

1. Ander I.P., Fuith L.C., Daxenbichler G., Marth C., Dapunt O.: Correlation between steroid hormone receptors, histological and clinical parameters in ovarian carcinoma, Gynecol. Obstet. Invest. 25: 135-140, 1988
2. Bizzi A., Codegoni A.M., Landoni F., Marelli G., Marsoni S., Spina A.M., Torri W., Mangioni C.: Steroid receptors in epithelial ovarian carcinoma: relation to clinical parameters and survival, Cancer Res. 48: 6222-6226, 1988
3. Harding M., Cowan S., Hole D., Cassidy L., Kitchener H., Davis J., Leake R.: Estrogen and progesterone receptors in ovarian cancer, Cancer 65: 486-491, 1990

4. Iacobelli S., Scambia G., Natoli C., Battaglia F., Polizzi G., Benedetti-Panici P., Baiocchi G., Perrone L., Mancuso S.: Steroid hormone receptors in human ovarian tumors, Conte P.F., Ragni N., Rosso R., Vermorken J.B. (Hrsg.): Multimodal treatment of ovarian cancer, New York: 11-26, 1989
5. Iversen O.E., Skaarland E., Utaaker E.: Steroid receptor content in human ovarian tumors: survival of patients with ovarian carcinoma related to steroid receptor content, Gynecol. Oncol. 23: 65-76, 1986
6. Kauppila A., Vierikko P., Kivinen S., Stenbäck F., Vihko R.: Clinical significance of estrogen and progestin receptors in ovarian cancer, Obstet. Gynecol. 61: 320-326, 1983
7. Kuhnel R., Delemarre J.F., Rao B.R., Stolk J.G.: Correlation of multiple steroid receptors with histological type and grade in human ovarian cancer, Int. J. Gynecol. Pathol. 6:248-256,1987
8. Kuhnel R., de Graaf J., Rao B.R., Stolk J.G.: Androgen receptor predominance in human ovarian carcinoma, J. Steroid Biochem. 26: 393-397, 1987
9. Masood S., Heitmann J., Nuss R.C., Benrubi G.I.: Clinical correlation of hormone receptor status in epithelial ovarian cancer, Gynecol. Oncol. 34: 57-60, 1989
10. Richman C.M., Holt J.A., Lorincz M.A., Herbst A.L.: Persistence and distribution of estrogen receptor in advanced epithelial ovarian carcinoma after chemotherapy, Obstet. Gynecol. 65: 257-263, 1985
11. Rose P.G., Reale F.R., Longcope C., Hunter R.E.: Prognostic significance of estrogen and progesterone receptors in epithelial ovarian cancer, Obstet. Gynecol. 76: 258-263, 1990
12. Rowland K., Bonomi P., Wilbanks G., Yordan E., Graham J., Dunne C.: Hormone receptors in ovarian carcinoma (meeting abstract), Proc. Am. Soc. Clin. Oncol. 4: 117, 1985
13. Schneider J., Edler L., Kleine W., Volm M.: DNA analysis chemoresistance testing and hormone receptor levels as prognostic factors in advanced ovarian carcinoma, Arch. Gynecol. Obstet. 248: 45-52, 1990
14. Schwartz P.E., Mac Lusky N., Merino M.J., Livolsi V.A., Kohorn E.I., Eisenfeld A.: Are cytosol estrogen and progestin receptors of prognostic significance in the management of epithelial ovarian cancers? Obstet. Gynecol. 68: 751-758, 1986
15. Slotman B.J., Kuhnel R., Rao B.R., Dijkhuizen G.H., de Graaf J., Stolk J.G.: Importance of steroid receptors and aromatase activity in the prognosis of ovarian cancer: high tumor progesterone receptor levels correlate with longer survival, Gyn. Onc. 33: 76-81, 1989
16. Spona J., Gitsch E., Salzer H., Karrer K.: Estrogen- and gestagen-receptors in ovarian carcinoma, Gynecol. Obstet. Invest. 16: 189-98, 1983
17. Sutton G.P., Senior M.B., Strauss J.F., Mikuta J.J.: Estrogen and progesterone receptors in epithelial ovarian malignancies, Gynecol. Oncol. 23: 176-82, 1986
18. Teufel G., Geyer H., de Gregorio G., Fuchs A., Kleine W., Pfleiderer A.: Östrogen- und Progesteronrezeptoren in malignen Ovarialtumoren, Geburtsh. u. Frauenheilk. 43: 732-740, 1983
19. Würz H., Wassner E., Citoler P., Schulz K.-D., Kaiser R.: Multiple cytoplasmic steroid hormone receptors in benign and malignant ovarian tumors and in disease-free ovaries, Tumor Diagnostik & Therapie 4:15-20, 1983

Cellular DNA Content as a New Prognostic Tool in Patients with Borderline Tumors of the Ovary. A Second Look

C.Tropé, J. Kærn, G. Kristensen, V. Abeler, E.O. Pettersen

Introduction

The over all survival of patients with ovarian borderline tumors has in several studies been reported as excellent, but a small fraction of patients, even in early stages, died of disease [1]. Stage of disease is a strong prognostic parameter but not of that importance as within frankly malignant neoplasms [2]. Histopathologic type and grade of differentiation are important prognostic factors in invasive carcinoma, with mucinous tumors doing better than the other types. Cellular atypia have been suggested of prognostic importance in borderline tumors [Russel 1984], but such grading is highly subjective and difficult to reproduce and standardize and not clearly related to the clinical outcome and therefore of limit value in prediction of individualized prognosis [3,4,5].

The histopathologic diagnosis of borderline tumors is difficult, and a true problem is that some pathologists do not accept borderline tumors as a separate diagnosis and therefore classify them as either benign or as invasive carcinoma. The distinction to clearly malignant tumors may be impossible but essential for selection of therapy and the prognosis of the patient.

The attitude to borderline tumors have become more conservative according to surgical approach allowing young patients to preserve their reproductive potential. Supporting this the need of more reproducible and objective prognostic parameters have become even more necessary.

In the last 2 decades nuclear DNA content have in several studies been shown to be of prognostic value in epithelial ovarian carcinoma [6,7]. Some of these studies have included borderline tumors, although only a small number of cases [8].

Abnormal DNA content measured by microspectrophotometry of Feulgen stained slides or by flow cytometry (FCM-DNA) have been associated with poor prognosis. A very few borderline tumors shows aneuploidy, but aneuploidy have been reported to indicate poor prognosis [9,10].

The aim of this retrospective study was to analyze the prognostic value of FCM-DNA ploidy in a large group of consecutive borderline patients with long-term follow-up treated in one institution, to improve the validity of our pilot study which showed that ploidy determinations might be a helpful tool in identifying the truly malignant borderline tumors [10].

Materials and Methods

Of 370 patients with ovarian borderline tumors treated at the Norwegian Radium Hospital from 1970 to June 1982 sections from formalin-fixed paraffin-embedded tissue from the primary tumor were accessible for flow cytometric DNA analysis in 335 cases. In 35 cases we did not succeed in getting hold of the paraffin-embedded blocks. The histopathological diagnosis was confirmed by one of us VA and sections from the area presenting most cellular atypia of the epithelial cell layers (avoiding inflammatory and necrotic cells) were selected for FCM-DNA. The paraffin-method described by Hedley et al.[11] with minor modifications [12,13] was used.

A laboratory built high-resolution flow cytometer [14] was used for measuring the nuclear DNA content. The use of external standards to perform a zero set of the multichannel analyzer and the ploidy definitions was as earlier described [10]. If only one G0/G1 peak was present the tumor was defined as diploid. If more than 1 peak, with exception of the diploid G2/M peak, were present the tumor was defined as aneuploid. Because of the relative poor resolution of the DNA histograms and the many pitfalls in calculation of S-phase within the paraffin-technique, we have not performed S-phase analysis. In 14 (4,2%) cases the DNA histograms were not evaluable for ploidy determination (»noise« and coefficient of variation >10%), leaving 321 diploid and aneuploid tumors, which is called the »ploidy-group«.

Histologic parameters as type, cellular atypia, tumor growth on the ovarian surface, tumor size, pseudomyxoma peritonei together with clinical parameters as age at diagnose, stage of disease inclusive ascites, surgical procedure, residual tumor after primary surgery, postoperative treatment and survival-data as relapse, localization of relapse, relapse-free period, cause of death and survival were registrated. Follow-up was complete and august 1991 was entered as the end point of the study. The follow-up data was collected from the medical records and the Cancer Registry of Norway.

Treatment

During the study period several different treatment protocols have been effective. Tumors of all stages have been treated in conformity with the protocols for invasive carcinomas. These protocols included surgery alone, adjuvant treatment with external pelvic radiotherapy or instillation of isotopes, and chemotherapy.

Statistical methods

Cancer-related survival was defined as the period from treatment in our institution to death of disease. Corrected (cancer related) survival rates was based on death from borderline malignancies only. The method of Kaplan and Meier [15] and the log-rank-test [16] was used to estimate and compare survival curves. The relation between the different prognostic variables were calculated with the F-test.

Results

Of 370 borderline tumors evaluable DNA-histograms were obtained in 321 cases. No statistical significant difference in any evaluated parameter, inclusive survival, were observed between the ploidy-group (n=321) (group A), the total group (n=370) (group B), the group without sample for FCM-ploidy examination (n=35) (group C) or the group with not evaluable FCM-DNA-histograms (n=14) (group D) (Table 1).

Of the evaluable DNA-histograms 293 were diploid (91,3%) and 28 were aneuploid (8,7%). The distribution of the analyzed histopathological and clinical parameters within the diploid and aneuploid groups are shown in Table 2. Statistical significant differences between the two groups was found concerning stage of disease ($p<0,0001$), histological types ($p=0,0096$), grade of atypia ($p<0,0001$), pseudomyxoma peritonei ($p<0,0001$), relapse ($p<0,0001$) and survival ($p<0,0001$). Within the diploid tumors 250 (85%) had stage I disease (64% stage IA) and only 43 (15%) were within stage II and III. In contrast 15 (54%) of the aneuploid tumors were within stage I disease (39% stage IA) and 13 (47%) had stage II and III ($p<0,001$).

Table 1: Patient characteristics in 370 ovarian borderline tumors treated at the Norwegian Radium Hospital between 1970-1982

		Group A n=321	Group B n=370	p-value	Group C n=35	p-value	Group D n=14	p-value
Age	<40	88	101		7		6	
	40-70	190	221	0,9838	25	0,3677	6	0,4148
	>70	43	48		3		2	
Stage	I	265	311		33		13	
	II	18	20	0,8527	1	0,1930	1	0,3897
	III	38	39		1		0	
Histol. type	mucinous	156	178		15		7	
	serous	149	174	0,9865	18	0,8161	7	0,6907
	other	16	18		2		0	
Atypia	mild	103	127		17		7	
	moderate	204	228	0,8253	17	0,1614	7	0,3292
	severe	14	5		1		0	
Tumor growth	no	255	297		31		11	
	yes	56	60	0,8818	3	0,3997	1	0,0636
	?	10	13		1		2	
Pseudo-myxoma	no	292	340		34		14	
	yes	29	30	0,7657	1	0,3530	0	0,4894
Tumor size	≤10cm	129	154	0,7604	15	0,9011	10	0,0408
	>10cm	192	216		20		4	
Residual tumor	no	315	364	0,9728	35	0,8710	14	0,6079
	yes	6	6		0		0	
Surgery	H+SBO+O	249	290	0,9756	28	0,9575	13	0,3051
	»less«	72	82		9		1	
Postop. treatment	no	79	89	0,9035	31	0,3512	10	0,9842
	yes	242	283		6		4	
Relapse	no	291	339		35	0,1165	13	0,8472
	yes	30	31	0,7546	0		1	
Survival	Alive	237	274		26		11	
	Dead OC	28	29	0,9018	0	0,1203	1	0,9246
	Dead ICD	56	67		9		2	

H+SBO+O = total hysterectomy; OC = ovarian carcinomas; ICD = intercurrent disease

Table 2: Ploidy in relation to classical prognostic factors

		Diploid n = 293		Aneuploid n = 28		P-value
Age	<40 40-70 >40	81 176 36		7 14 7		0,1664
Stage	IA IB IC	187 44 19	250	11 2 2	15	
	IIA IIB	2 13	15	0 3	3	0,0001
	III	28		10		
Histologic type	serous mucinous endometrioid clearcell mixed unclass	142 139 5 2 5 0	12	7 17 1 0 2 1	4	0,0723 0,0096
Atypia	mild moderate severe	96 189 8		7 15 6		<0,0001
Tumorsize cm	≤10 >10	120 173		9 19		0,4796
Tumor growth on the ovarian surface	no yes ?	236 48 9		19 8 1		0,2576
Pseudomyxoma peritonei (mucinous tumor)	no yes	119 20		8 9		0,0004
Residual tumor	no yes	289 4		26 2		0,1537
Surgical procedure in patients without residual tumor	H+BSO+O USO BSO H+BSO BSO+O	227 13 13 29 7	62	22 0 0 3 1	4	0,9170
Postop. adjuvant treatment in patients without residual tumor	no Ext Isotope Thiotepa Ext+Iso Ext+Thio Iso+Thio	77 49 64 39 28 6 26	212	2 7 5 6 3 2 1	24	0,0575

Cont. table 2

		Diploid n = 293	Aneuploid n = 28	P-value
Relapse	no	280	11	<0,0001
	yes	13	17	
Survival	alive	228	7	
	dead of disease	11	17	<0,0001
	dead of ICD	52	4	

H+BSO+O = Hysterectomy + bilateral salpingo oophorectomy + omenectomy
USO = Salpingo oophorectomy unilateralis
BSO = Salpingo oophorectomy
H+BSO= Hysterectomy + bilateral salpingo oophorectomy
BSO+O = Bilateral salpingo oophorectomy + omenectomy
EXT = External radiotherapy
EXT+ISO = External radiotherapy + isotope
EXT+THIO = External radiotherapy + Thiotepa
ISO+THIO = Isotope + Thiotepa
ICD = Intercurrent disease

Regarding histological type, there was a tendency towards more aneuploid tumors in the mucinous group than in the serous group but not statistically significant (p=0,07), but other histologic types (endometrioid, mixed and clearcell tumors) made up 14% of the aneuploid tumors compared to 4% of the diploid tumors (p=0,009). Severe atypia was more frequently observed in the aneuploid tumors (21%) compared to the diploid tumors (3%), p<0,0001. In the mucinous tumors pseudomyxoma peritonei was present in 14% of the diploid compared to 53% of the aneuploid tumors (p=0,0004). Presence of pseudomyxoma were significally more frequently in advanced stages of the disease. Tumor growth on the ovarian surface within the diploid tumors was significally more frequent in the serous tumors compared to the mucinous tumors (p=0,03); but among the aneuploid tumors, tumor growth was equally distributed between the serous (33%) and mucinous (35%) tumors.

Tumorsize correlated to histologic type. Tumors larger than 10 cm was present in 79% of the mucinous tumors and in 41% of the serous only (p<0,0001). No statistically significant difference in tumor size (>10cm) was found within the mucinous tumors between diploid tumors and aneuploid tumors. In the serous tumors there was a tendency although statistically not significant towards large tumors in the aneuploid groups. Only 6 patients had residual tumor after primary surgery. Four were diploid and 2 were aneuploid tumors. In 249 patients radical surgery consisted of H+BSO+O (227 had diploid tumors and 22 had aneuploid tumor). More conservative surgery was performed in 66 patients. Of these, 62 had diploid tumors (13 had unilateral adnexextirpation, 13 BSO, 29 H+BSO and 7 BSO+O). Three aneuploid tumor patients in stage IIB had H+BSO and 1 patient in stage III had BSO+O (table 2).

Postoperative treatment

The 6 patients with residual tumor all received postoperative treatment, either external irradiation or thiotepa or a combination of these treatment modalities.

Of the tumorfree operated patients 236 (75%) received adjuvant postoperative treatment, 212 diploid and 24 aneuploid. Seventy-nine (25%) were treated with surgery alone, 77 diploid and 2 aneuploid. The number of deaths in the different postoperative treatments-groups in relation to ploidy are shown in table 2. As can be seen there were no difference in survival between the different postoperative treatments groups.

Only 30 of the 321 patients relapsed (9,3%) and of these 28 died of disease (8,7%) (table 2). There was no differences between diploid and aneuploid tumors concerning relapse-localization. In the diploid group 13 patients relapsed (4,4%) of which 11 died of disease (3,8%). The 2 relapse-patients were alive NED after treatment were so for 104 and 105 months, respectively. In the group of patients with aneuploid tumor 17 relapsed and all died of disease (60,7%) (table 2). This difference in cancer-related survival (CRS) between diploid and aneuploid tumor patients was highly statistical significant, p<0,0001. Crude survival rate in the diploid group was 75,0% compared to 21,5% in the aneuploid group, p<0,0001.

Four of the 6 patients with residual tumor died of disease. Two had diploid tumor, one stage IIB-serous, the other stage III mucinous, and 2 had aneuploid tumors, both stage III mucinous. The two patients who are alive with residual tumor have survived for 240 and 108 months, respectively. Both had diploid tumors and stage III disease (one serous treated with extern irradiation and one mucinous tumor treated with thiotepa).

Of the tumorfree operated patients who died of disease 9 had diploid and 15 aneuploid tumors. Within the diploid group 3 had stage IA disease (2 mucinous and 1 endometrioid), 1 stage IIB (serous) and 5 stage III disease (3 serous and 2 mucinous). All were operated with H+BSO+O, except from one (st IA, mucinous), who had H+BSO only. Two did not receive postoperative adjuvant treatment (one: stage IA-mucinous; and one stage III-mucinous). In the aneuploid group 5 had stage IA (3 mucinous,1 mixed tumor and 1 with unclassificabel histologic type). 3 had stage IIB (2 mucinous and 1 serous) and 7 had stage III (5 mucinous, 1 serous and 1 endometrioid). Eleven patients were operated with H+BSO+O; in 3 patients omentectomy was not performed (2 stage IIB and I stage III) and in 1 patients hysterectomy was not done (stage IIB). All 15 received postoperative adjuvant treatment.

The classical prognostic factors showed to be important for survival [10], but ploidy is a much stronger prognostic factor. Figures 1ab, 2ab, 3ab, 4ab, 5ab show survival curves comparing classical prognostic factors (A) like stage of disease (fig. 1), histologic types (fig. 2), cellular atypia (fig. 3) surgical procedure (fig. 4) and age of diagnosis (fig. 5) with survival curves where ploidy (B) is added to these classical prognostic factors. As can be clearly seen adding ploidy to the classical prognostic factors divides the patients into real high and low risk patients in a significant better way than the classical prognostic factors alone. Mainly all patients with stage IA diploid tumors survive but only 50% of the patients with stage IA aneuploid tumors survive (fig. 2c).

In the diploid stage I group of patients both the 76 patients who did not receive adjuvant treatment and the 176 patients who received adjuvant treatment had a CRS of 99%. The only one patients with diploid tumor and advanced disease who did not receive postoperative treatment died of disease. The 38 diploid patients with advanced disease and postoperative treatment showed CRS of 85%.

Of the patients with aneuploid tumor only one patient in stage I (alive NED) and one patient in stage III (death of disease) did not receive adjuvant treatment. Concerning the aneuploid-tumorfree-patients who received adjuvant treatment, 14 patients in stage I had a CRS of 58% and 10 patients in stage II/III had a CRS of 10%. In the treated group of patients the aneuploid tumors showed a poor survival compared to the diploid both within stage I patients, $p<0,0001$ and within stage II/III patients, $p<0,0001$ (fig. 1b). The same tendency can be seen when stratifying for ploidy in the different histology groups, all the aneuploid groups showed statistical poorer survival than the diploid groups $p<0,0001$ (fig. 2a,b). Cellular atypia was not found to be of prognostic value, but compared to the diploid tumors within the aneuploid tumors severe atypia was significantly more frequent and when stratifying for ploidy all aneuploid tumors independent of grade of atypia had statistical significant poorer survival compared to the diploid tumors, $p<0,0001$ (fig. 3a,b).

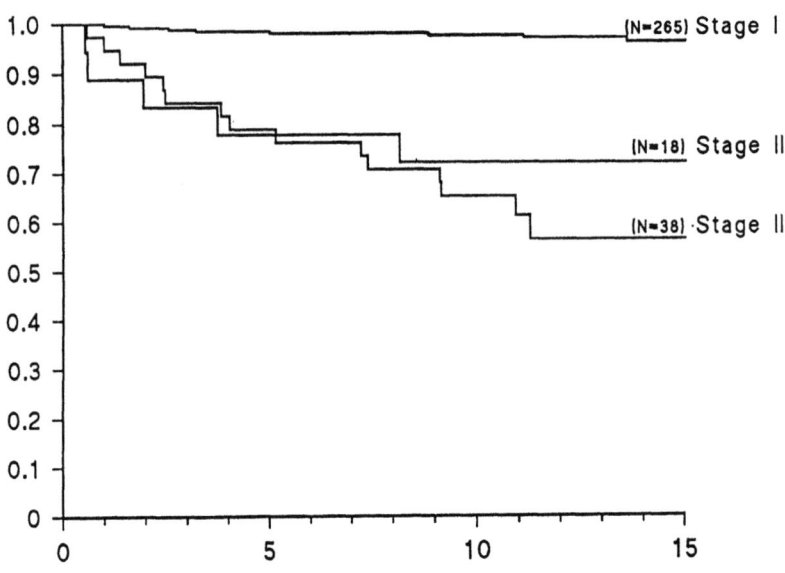

Fig. 1a: Borderline ovarian tumors 1970-1982; 15 years corrected survival in relation to stage

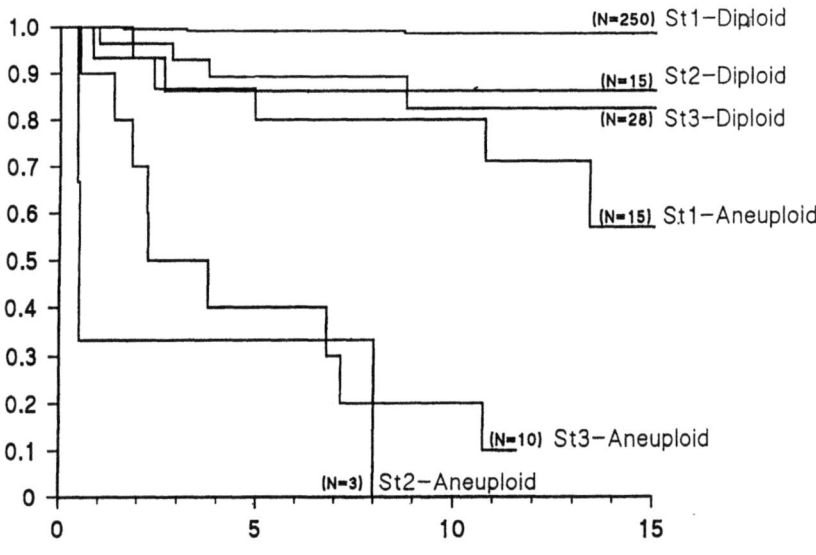

Fig. 1b: Borderline ovarian tumors 1970-1982; corrected survival in relation to stage and ploidy

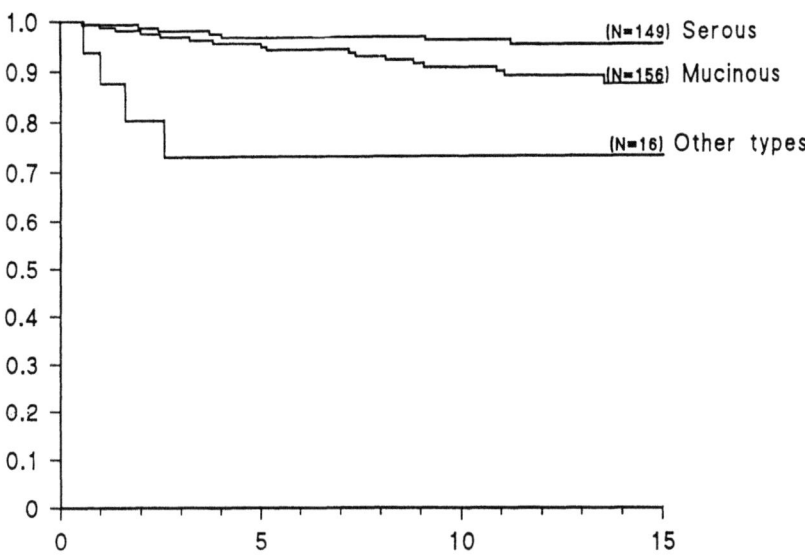

Fig. 2a: Borderline ovarian tumors 1970-1982; 15 years corrected survival in relation to histologic type

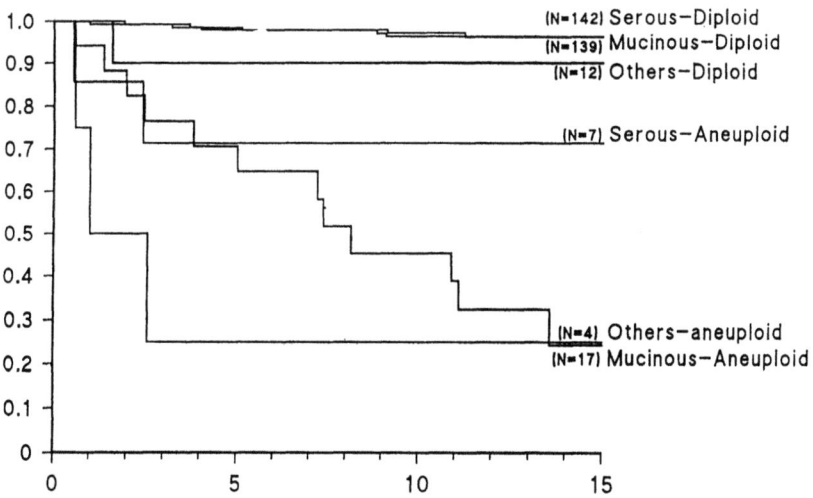

Fig. 2b: Borderline ovarian tumors 1970-1982; 15 years corrected survival in relation to ploidy and histologic type

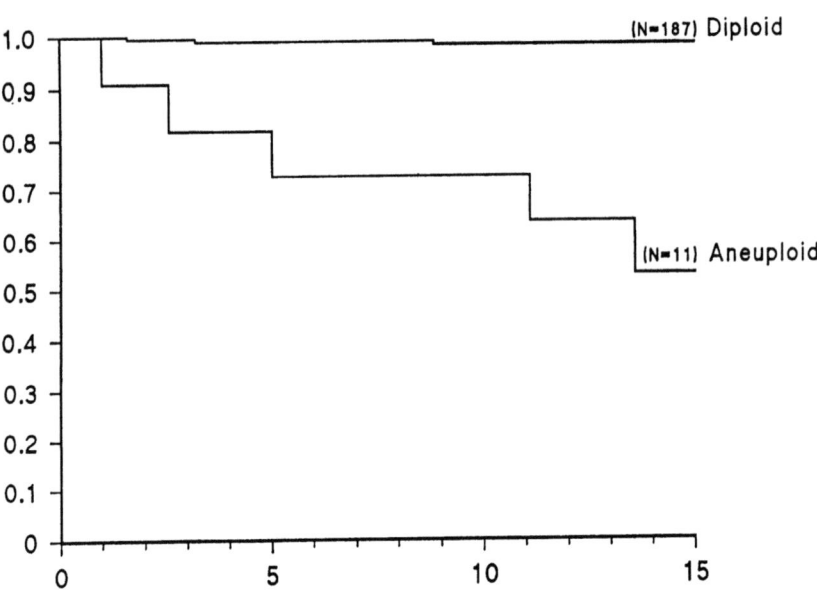

Fig. 2c: Borderline ovarian tumors 1970-1982; 15 years corrected survival in relation to ploidy in stage IA patients

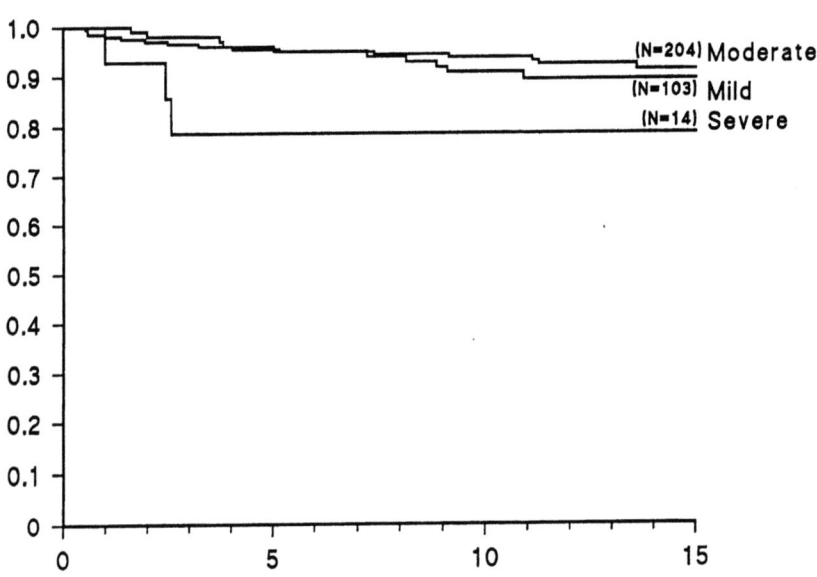

Fig. 3a: Borderline ovarian tumors 1970-1982; 15 years corrected survival in relation to cellular atypia

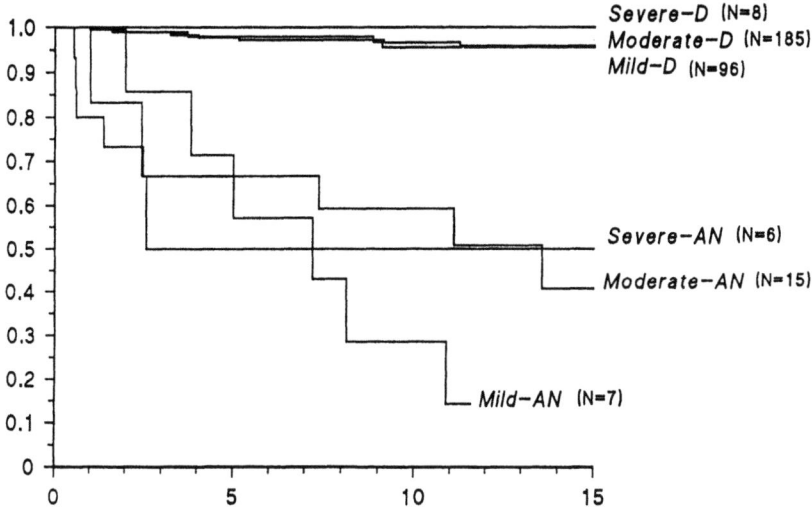

Fig. 3b: Borderline ovarian tumors 1970-1982; 15 years corrected survival in relation to cellular atypia and ploidy

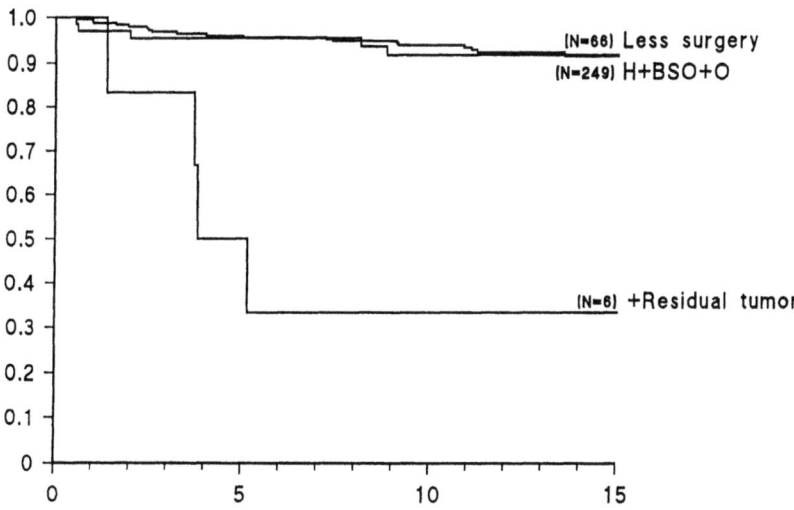

Fig. 4a: Borderline ovarian tumors 1970-1982; 15 years corrected survival in relation to residual tumor and surgical procedure

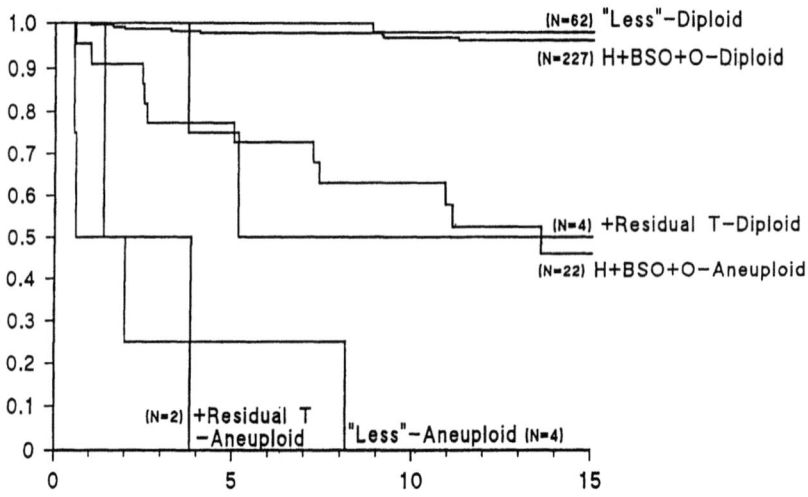

Fig. 4b: Borderline ovarian tumors 1970-1982; 15 years corrected survival in relation to ploidy, residual tumor and surgical procedure

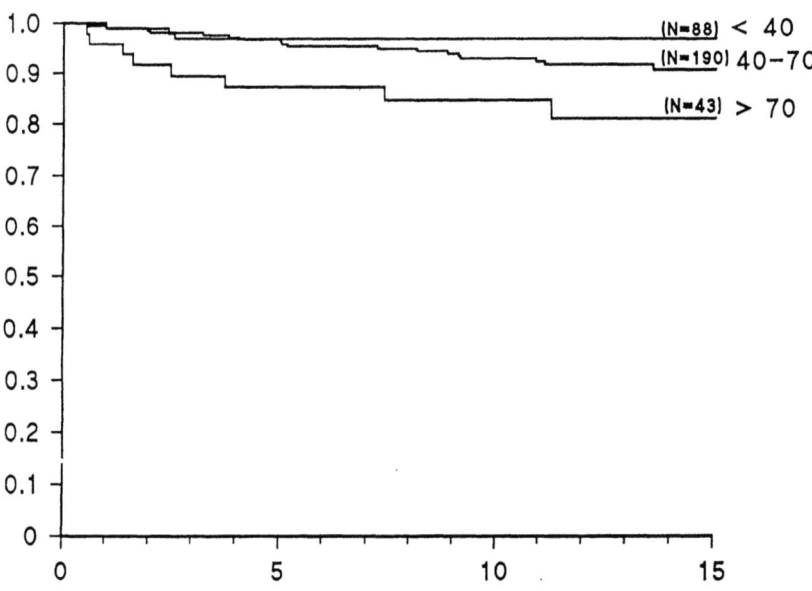

Fig. 5a: Borderline ovarian tumors 1970-1982; 15 years corrected survival in relation to age

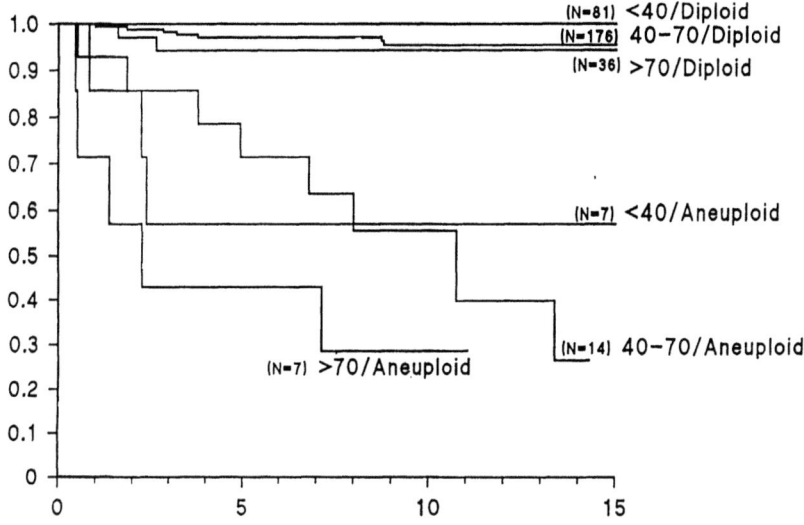

Fig. 5b: Borderline ovarian tumors 1970-1982; corrected survival in relation to age and ploidy

Table 3: Postoperative treatment in 315 radical operated tumorfree patients with ovarian borderline tumors

	Diploid number	DOD	Aneuploid number	DOD	Total number	DOD
No	77	2	2	1	79	3
Ext	49	3	7	5	56	8
Isotope	64	1	5	2	69	3
Thiotepa	39	1	6	5	45	6
Ext+^{198}Au	28	0	3	1	31	1
Ext+Thiotepa	6	1	2	1	8	2
Isotope+Thiotepa	26	1	1	0	27	1

EXT = External radiotherapy; Isotope = ^{32}P / ^{198}AU; DOD = Dead of disease

Table 4: Characteristics of patients (n=7) alive with aneuploid tumor

	1	2	3	4	5	6	7
Age	61	60	31	53	34	70	38
Stage	IA	IA	IA	IB	IB	IC	III
Histologic type	M	M	S	S	S	S	M
Surgery	all patiens: H+BSO+O						
Adj. treatment	No	^{198}Au	Ext	No	^{32}P	Ext+Thio	^{32}P+Thio
Survival	174	194	219	184	121	136	166
FCM - C value	3,1	3,7	3,5	3,5	2,8	2,5	3,4

M = mucinous; S = serous; H+BSO+O = Hysterectomy + bilateral salphingo oophorectomy + omenectomy; Ext.+Thio = External radiotherapy + Thiotepa; Ext.= External radiotherapy; Thio = Thiotepa

Table 5: The cause of death in relation to observation time and ploidy

Year	Alive			Dead of disease			Dead of intercurrent disease		
	T	D	A	T	D	A	T	D	A
2	305	283	22	9	3	6	7	7	0
5	291	273	18	16	6	10	14	14	0
10	271	258	13	24	10	14	26	25	1
15	246	238	8	28	11	17	47	44	3
Observation time 1/8-91	237	230	7	28	11	17	51	47	4

T = Total; D = Diploid; A = Aneuploid

Patients left with residual tumor after primary surgery showed a significant poorer prognosis than tumorfree operated patients, p<0,0001. No statistical significant difference was found between the group of tumorfree patients operated with H+BSO+O and those operated with minor surgical procedure (fig. 4a). Again when stratifying for ploidy tumorfree patients with diploid tumors had a significant better survival than patients with aneuploid tumors (fig. 4) (table 3). Age at diagnose have earlier been shown to be of prognostic value (<40 / 40-70 / >70 years). Again when stratified for ploidy all patients with aneuploid tumor showed poor prognosis compared to the patients with diploid tumor, p<0,0001 (fig. 5a,b).

At the end point of the study 237 patients (73,7%) were alive NED, 230 diploid (included the 2 relapse-patients) and 7 of the aneuploid tumor. Of these aneuploid patients 6 were within stage I (3 stage IA, 2 stage IB and 1 stage IC) and 1 within stage III, 4 had serous tumors and 2 mucinous, (1 stage IA and 1 stage III). All 7 had H+BSO+O. Except 1 patient (stage IA, mucinous) all had received adjuvant postoperative treatment. The DNA-index of these 7 patients did not differ from the total aneuploid group (c-value : 2,5-3,7) (table 4). The cause of death in relation to observation time and ploidy is shown in table 5.

Univariate analysis within the ploidy group showed that ploidy, stage of disease, residual tumor, histologic type, pseudomyxoma peritonei, tumor growth on the ovarian surface, tumor size and age at diagnosis were of important prognostic value (table 6).

All 15 aneuploid stage I patients were operated with H+BSO+O. Patients in stage I and diploid, operated with H+BSO+O had CRS of 99% compared to 62% for the aneuploid. Less aggressive operated stage I diploid patients had CRS of 98%; including all stages (tumorfree) the correspondent figure was also 98% (only 3 patients with advanced disease and diploid tumor had minor surgery than H+BSO+O, all 3 alive NED). Four aneuploid patients in advanced stage (tumorfree) with minor surgery all died of disease (fig. 6).

Table 6: Univariate analysis in the total group of patients (n=321) with ovarian borderline tumors. 15 years corrected survival

Factor		CHI-square	p-value
Ploidy	diploid aneuploid	136,4	<0,0001
Stage	I II III	71,94	<0,0001
Pseudo- myxoma	no yes	39,15	<0,0001
Residual tumor	no yes	38,05	<0,0001
Extra capsular growth	no yes	9,87	0,0017
Histologic type	serous mucinous other	9,92	0,0016
Age	<40 40-70 >70	9,09	0,0029
Tumorsize in cm	≤10 >10	6,57	0,0104
Isotop	no yes	6,40	0,0114
External irradiation	no yes	5,06	0,0245
Thiotepa	no yes	3,32	0,0685
Postoperative treatment	no yes	3,08	0,0793
Surgical procedure	H+BSO+O »less«	2,48	0,1150
Grade of atypia	mild moderate severe	0,26	0,6133

log likelihood = - 157,7028
* in 10 patients no information on this parameter
H+BSO+O = Hysterectomy + bilateral salphingo oophorectomy + omenectomy
»less« = USO, BSO, BSO+H, BSO+O
Postoperative treatment = No or Isotp, External irradiation and Thiotepa as single therapy or in a combination

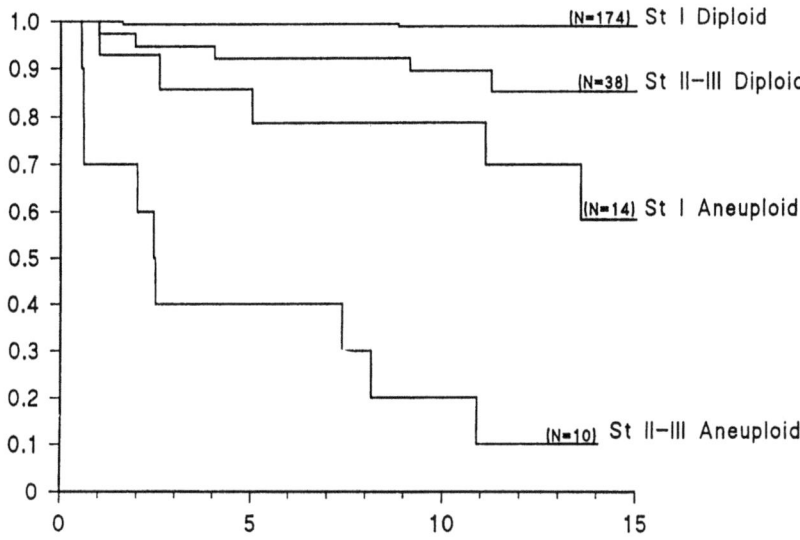

Fig. 6: Borderline ovarian tumors 1970-1982; 15 years corrected survival in relation to stage and ploidy in patients without residual tumor and with adjuvant treatment

Discussion

The present retrospective study including 370 consecutive patients with ovarian borderline lesions with complete follow up of at least 9 years and a median of 127 months had previously been analyzed by Cox regression multivariate analysis concerning the different classical prognostic variables in regard to cancer related survival (dead of disease) FIGO stage, followed by histology type were the most important significant prognostic indicators of survival. Age was of prognostic value only concerning long-term survival. No benefit occurred from postoperative adjuvant treatment [17]. We identified a high risk group of patients with borderline tumor as: above the age of 60 and mucinous tumor, stage II or III. According to our previously findings such patient had an established chance of long term survival of approximately 75%. Although it is quite clear that tumors of borderline malignancy have a much better prognosis than frankly invasive carcinoma their biologic behavior has caused many controversies. Even patients with stage I disease may relapse but often after a relapsefree period of 10 to 15 years. Tumors that show dissemination to an extent that life of the patient is threatened are undoubtedly best classified as cancers. Compared to poorly differentiated ovarian cystadenocarcinoma the borderline tumors may behave less aggressively, never the less the prognosis of these patients is far from optimal. When dividing patients into high or low risk groups we are at the moment using quite subjective clinical and histopathological criteria. To increase our armentarium objectively we have used cellular DNA content as a new prognostic factor and we have shown in a pilot study that patients with aneuploid tumors regardless of histology and stage had a less than 40% chance of long term survival. Ploidy therefore seemed to be a superior prognostic factor in patients with borderline tumors [10]. In the present study where we have analyzed the total material of borderline tumors treated at the Norwegian Radium Hospital between 1970-1982. DNA ploidy was found to be the strongest independent predictor of the clinical outcome (table 5). Of the evaluable histograms 293 were diploid 91,3% and only 28 were aneuploid 8,7%. Aneuploidy is related to histology and mucinous endometrioid and clearcell tumors were found to have a worse prognosis than serous tumors. Twentyfive percent of the endometrioid / clearcell and 11 percent of the mucinous were aneuploid in contrast to 6% of the serous tumors. Ploidy also showed a correlation to stage of the disease. Thirtyseven percent of stage III tumors were aneuploid compared to 10% within the diploid tumors. No differences in survival was found between the groups of patients who received postoperative treatment. The addition of postoperative treatment was not found to influence survival neither within the diploid tumors or the aneuploid tumors. Univariate analysis showed that ploidy, stage of disease, residual tumor, histologic type, pseudomyxoma peritonei, tumorgrowth on the ovarian surface, tumorsize and age at diagnosis were of important prognostic values. This results support our pilot study and previous studies using either flow cytometry or absorption cytometry [8,18-20]. Patients with diploid tumors showed independent of the classical prognostic factors a significant better survival than the aneuploid tumors. (fig. 1ab, 2ab, 3ab, 4ab, 5ab).

The prognosis of diploid borderline tumors is so benign that there have been an enormous overtreatment and we would postulate that tumorfree surgery in diploid tumors is sufficient on the assumption of a properly staging procedure and assuring representative biopsy taken for nuclear DNA measurements. The biology of the aneuploid tumors corresponds that of frankly malignant carcinoma, so we suggest the term »low grade malignancy« to be reserved to the diploid tumors and consider the aneuploid tumors in the category of invasive carcinoma. Prospective randomized studies would be necessary to evaluate the possible positive influence of survival of postoperative adjuvant modern chemotherapy or modern radiotherapy in aneuploid borderline tumors and early invasive carcinoma.

Our conclusion is in agreement with that of Friedlander et al. [18] that DNA is the most important prognostic factor in patients with borderline tumors and must be included together with the classical prognostic factors in the future in the evaluation of the clinical outcome of the individual patient and in the stratification of treatment regimen. We mean that ploidy determination is a helpful tool in identifying the truely malignant borderline tumor.

At our institution we now after carefully staging use ploidy in a prospective study to define patients whom conservative treatment is justified. Conservative therapy is indicated in patients with stage IA diploid disease who desire to remain fertility. Standard treatment in all other good prognosis patients should be total hysterectomy plus bilateral salpingo-oophorectomy plus omentectomy with long-term follow up. Stage I aneuploid borderline disease are in our institution after radical surgery randomized to no postoperative treatment versus postoperative treatment with 6 courses of Paraplatine. To find out if adjuvant chemotherapy with our must effective single drug in ovarian cancer will increase the survival in the high risk patients.

References

1. Bostwick D.G., Tazelaar H.D., Ballon S.C., Hendrickson M.R., Kempson R.L.: Ovarian epithelial tumors of borderline malignancy: A clinical and pathologic study of 109 cases. Cancer 58: 2052-2065, 1986
2. Fox H., Burghardt E.: Prognostic indices in ovarian tumours of borderline malignancy with particular reference to morphometric analysis. In: Ovarian cancer by Tattersall M.H.: 69-101, 1988
3. Russell P.: The pathological assesments of ovarian neoplasms II. The prolifering epithelial tumours. Pathology 11: 259-282, 1979
4. Fox H.: Ovarian tumors of borderline malignancy. Progress in Cancer Research and Therapy 24: 137-150, 1983
5. Baak J.P.A., Fox H., Langley F.A., Buckley C.H.: The prognostic value of morphometry in ovarian epithelial tumors of borderline malignancy. Int. J. Gynecol. Path. 4: 186-191, 1985
6. Friedlander M.L., Taylor I.W., Russell P., Musgrove E.A., Hedley D.H., Tattersall M.H.N.: Ploidy as a prognostic factor in ovarian cancer. Int. J. Gynecol. Path. 2: 55-63, 1983
7. Rodenburg C.J., Cornelisse C.J., Heintz P.A.M., Hermans J., Fleuren G.J.: Tumor ploidy as a major prognostic factor in advanced ovarian cancer. Cancer 59: 317-323, 1987

8. Kühn W., Kaufmann M., Feichter G.E., Rummel H.H., Schmid H., Heberling D.: DNA flow cytometry, clinical and morphological parameters as prognostic factors for advanced malignant and borderline ovarian tumors. Gynecol. Oncol. 33: 360-367, 1989
9. Klemi P.J., Joensuu H., Kilholma P., Mäenpää J.: Clinical significance of abnormal nuclear DNA content in serous ovarian tumors. Cancer 62: 2005-2010, 1988
10. Kærn J., Tropé C., Kjorstad K.E., Abeler V., Pettersen E.O.: Cellular DNA content as a new prognostic tool in patients with borderline tumors of the ovary. Gynecol. Oncol. 38: 452-457, 1990
11. Hedley D.W., Friedlander M.L.. Taylor I.W., Rugg C.A., Musgrove E.A.: Method for analysis of cellular DNA content of paraffin embedded pathological material using flow cytometry. J. Histochem. Cytochem. 31: 1333-1335, 1983
12. Fosså S.D., Thorud E., Shoaib M.C., Pettersen E.O., Hoie J., Scott-Knudsen O.: DNA flow cytometry in primary breast carcinoma. Acta. Pathol. Microbiol. Immunol. Scand. Sect. 92: 475-480, 1984
13. Fosså S.D., Shoaib M.C., Pettersen E.O., Thorud E.: DNA flow cytometry of cells obtained from old paraffin embedded specimens. A comparison with results of scanning absorption cytometry. Pathol. Res. Pract. 181: 200-205, 1986
14. Lindmo T., Steen H.B.: Characteristics of a simple high resolution flow cytometry based on a flow configuration. Biophys. J. 28: 33-44, 1979
15. Kaplan E.L., Meier P.: Nonparametric estimation from incomplete observations. J. Am. Stat. Assoc. 53: 457-481, 1958
16. Tarone R.E., Ware J.: On distribution-free tests for equality of survival distributions. Biometrika 64: 156-160, 1977
17. Kærn J., Tropé C., Abeler V.M.: A retrospective study of 370 borderline tumors of the ovary treated at The Norwegian Radium Hospital 1970-1982: A review of clinicopathological features and treatment modalities. Submitted 1991
18. Friedlander M.L., Russel P., Taylor I.W., Hedley D.W. Tattersall M.H.N.: Flow cytometric analysis of cellular DNA content as an adjunct to the diagnosis of ovarian tumours of borderline malignancy. Path.: 301-306, 1984
19. Erhardt K., Auer G., Björkholm E. et al.: Prognostic significance of nuclear DNA content in serous ovarian. Cancer Research 44: 2198-2202, 1984
20. Dietel M., Arps H., Rohlff A., Bodecker R., Niendorf A.: Nuclear DNA content of borderline tumors of the ovary: correlation with histology and significance for prognosis. Virchows Arch. (Pathol. Anat.) 409: 829-836, 1986

Die flowzytometrische Bestimmung des nukleären DNA-Gehaltes bei malignen epithelialen Tumoren der Ovarien

J. Pfisterer[1], F. Kommoss[1], H. Renz[1], W. Sauerbrei[2], H.-G. Meerpohl[1], G. Teufel[1], A. Pfleiderer[1]

Eines der charakteristischen Merkmale maligner Ovarialtumoren ist ihre tumorbiologische Heterogenität, die von relativ benige verlaufenden Borderline-Tumoren auf der einen Seite bis zu hoch malignen, aggressiv metastasierenden Tumoren mit kurzer Überlebenszeit auf der anderen Seite reicht. Dieses breite klinische Spektrum ist mit klassischen morphologischen Kriterien und klinisch evaluierbaren prognostischen Faktoren nur teilweise beschreibbar, was zum Teil auch an der Subjektivität bei der Erhebung dieser Daten liegt, denkt man beispielsweise nur an die Festlegung des »postoperativen Tumorrestes« im Rahmen der Primäroperation. So liegt es nahe, nach einem Faktor zu suchen, der rasch und objektiv, jederzeit auch von anderen Untersuchern aus dem gleichen Material reproduzierbar, Aussagen über den weiteren klinischen Verlauf bei einer individuellen Patientin zuläßt.

Wir stellten uns deshalb die Frage, welche prognostische Bedeutung der nucleäre DNA-Gehalt besitzt, ob eine prognostische Bedeutung der proliferativen Aktivität vorliegt, hier gemessen als Relativprozent der sich in der S-Phase befindlichen Zellen. Weiterhin interessierte uns eine mögliche Korrelation dieser Faktoren mit traditionell etablierten prognostischen Faktoren wie Stadium, histologischem Grading oder dem Tumorrest nach cytoreduktiver chirurgischer Therapie. Ferner sollte geklärt werden, ob sich unter Zuhilfenahme dieser Parameter Patientinnen in prognostische Gruppen einteilen lassen, möglicherweise gar mit therapeutischen Konsequenzen.

In einer retrospektiven Analyse untersuchten wir insgesamt 226 nicht vorbehandelte Ovarialkarzinome der Stadien I bis IV, Ausschlußkriterien waren das Vorliegen eines oder mehrerer der folgenden Parameter: Nichtepitheliale maligne Ovarialtumoren, Borderline-Tumoren, Malignome anderer Entität in der

---

[1] Universitätsfrauenklinik Freiburg
[2] Institut für Medizinische Biometrie und Medizinische Informatik der Universität Freiburg

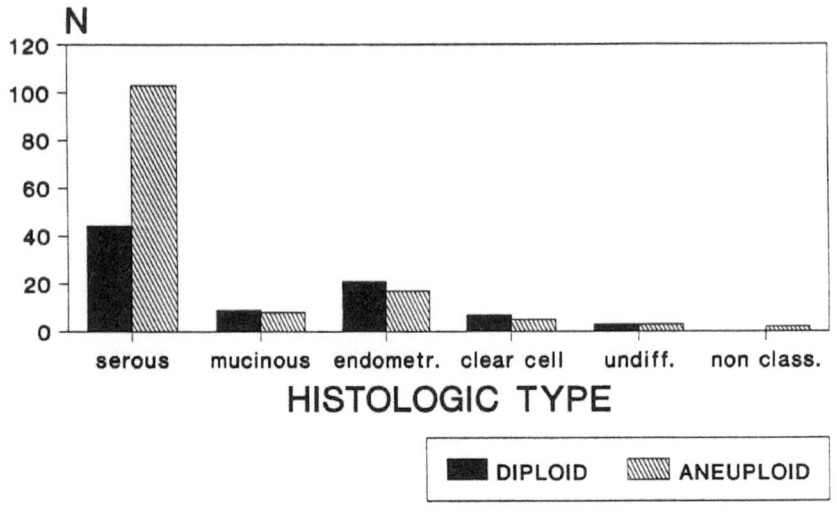

Abb. 1: Ploidy - histologic typ; stage I-IV

Anamnese, im Stadium III und IV nach der operativen Therapie eine andere Behandlung als eine Chemotherapie. Es lag folgende Stadienverteilung vor: FIGO I und II n=21, FIGO III n=141, FIGO IV n=64. Paraffin eingebettes Material wurde nach der leicht modifizierten Methode nach Hedley [1] aufgearbeitet und flowcytometrisch analysiert. Die S-Phase als Maß der proliferativen Aktivität wurde nur bei diploiden Tumoren in die Auswertung mit aufgenommen, da keines der erhältlichen Computerprogramme bei aneuploiden, sich überlappenden Populationen, zuverlässig die S-Phase berechnen kann. Das mediane Follow-up der Überlebenden betrug 36 Monate.

Betrachtet man die Ploidieverteilung hinsichtlich des histologischen Typs kann man erkennen, daß bei allen Tumoren außer den serösen das Verhältnis diploid zu aneuploid etwa 1:1 ist, bei den serösen jedoch finden sich signifikant häufiger aneuploide Tumoren (Abb. 1). Im Stadium I und II finden sich ebenfalls etwa gleich viel diploide wie aneuploide Tumoren, in den höheren Stadien überwiegen die aneuploiden, wobei, was für die spätere Analyse der Überlebenszeit wichtig ist, zwischen Stadium III und IV kein signifikanter Unterschied besteht (Abb. 2).

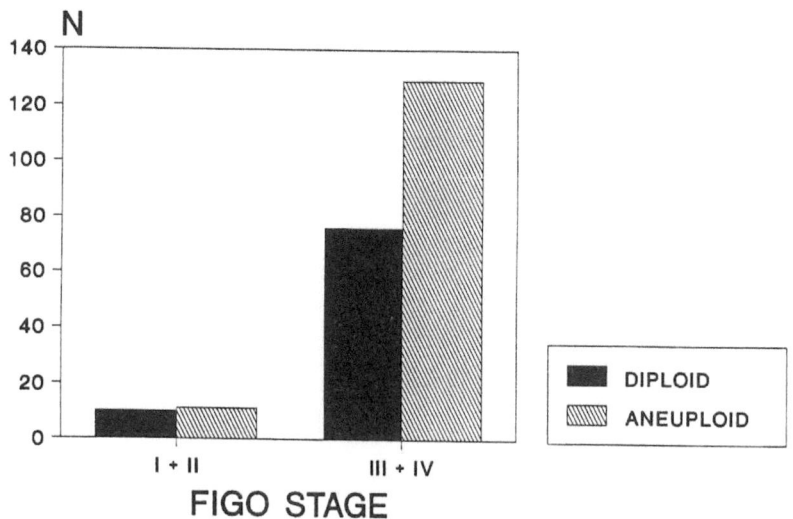

Abb. 2: Stadium - Ploidie; Stadium III vs Stadium IV: n.s.

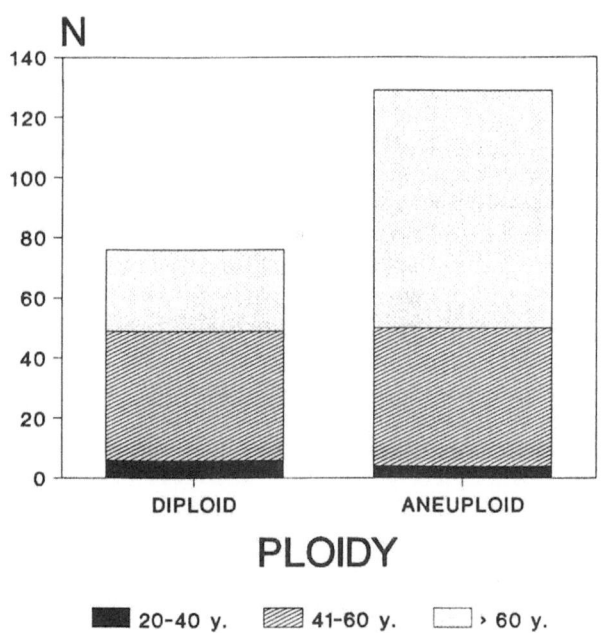

Abb. 3: Ploidie - Alter; Stadium III + IV; < 60 versus > 60 Jahre: p<0,001

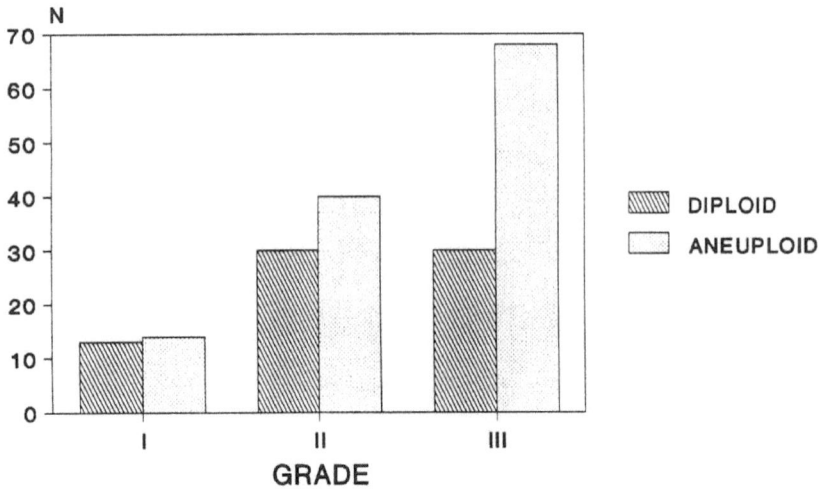

Abb. 4: Grading - ploidy; stage III+IV; G1 versus G2/G3: n.s.

Was die frühen Stadien anbelangt waren von den Patientinnen mit diploiden Tumoren nach 3 Jahren follow up 2 von 10 verstorben, von denen mit aneuploiden 4 von 11. Weitere Aussagen zu diesen Stadien sind aufgrund der geringen Fallzahl nicht sinnvoll. Betrachtet man im Stadium III und IV das Vorkommen von Tumoren mit diploiden und aneuploiden Stammlinien unter Berücksichtigung des Alters, so finden sich bei jüngeren Patientinnen gleich häufig diploide und aneuploide Tumoren, bei den über 60-jährigen liegen in der Mehrzahl aneuploide Tumoren vor, dies ist ein möglicher Faktor, der die mit zunehmendem Lebensalter schlechtere Prognose erklären könnte (Abb. 3).

Was das histologische Grading anbelangt, ist eine Zunahme von aneuploiden Tumoren zu finden, je geringer differenziert der Tumor ist (Abb. 4). Auch der Tumorrest nach cytoreduktiver Chirurgie scheint in Zusammenhang mit dem DNA-Gehalt zu stehen: Patientinnen, die sich auf einen Tumorrest kleiner 0,5 cm operieren ließen, hatten überwiegend diploide Tumoren, bei den anderen fanden sich zum überwiegenden Teil aneuploide (Abb. 5). Kein Zusammenhang mit der Ploidie konnte beim Ansprechen eines Tumors auf die durchgeführte Chemotherapie gefunden werden.

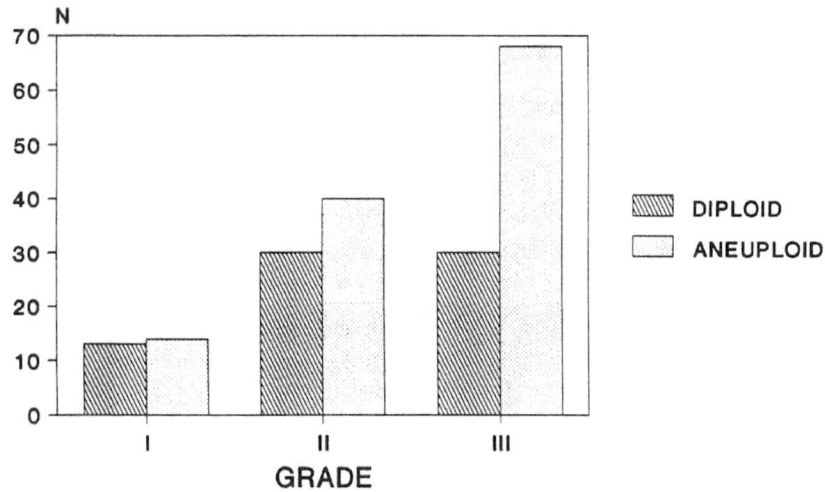

Abb. 5: Ploidie - postop. Tumorrest; Stadium III+IV

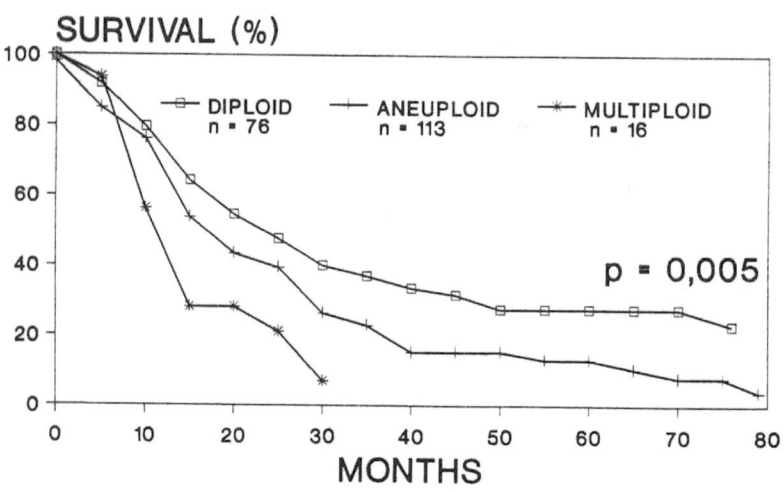

Abb. 6: Ploidie - Überleben; Stadium III+IV

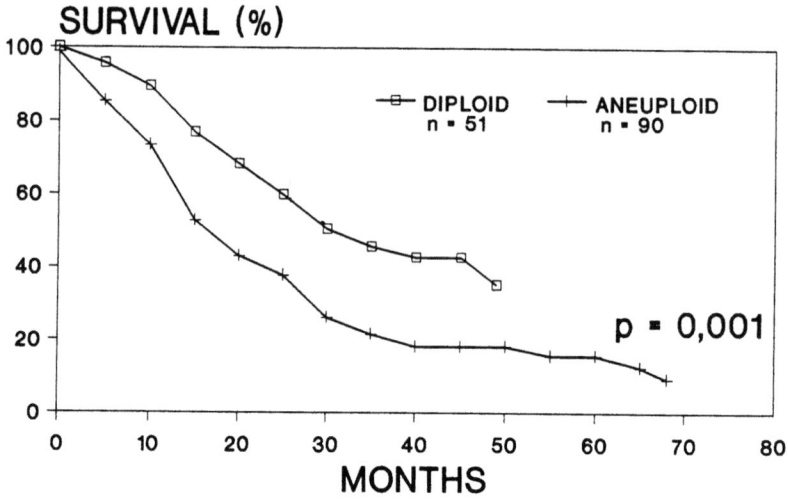

Abb. 7: Ploidie - Überleben; Stadium III

In den nach Kaplan-Meier geschätzten Überlebenskurven erkennt man, daß Patientinnen mit aneuploiden Tumoren signifikant kürzer überleben, als Sondergruppe mit besonders schlechter Prognose diejenigen mit sogenannten multiploiden Tumoren, d.h. mit mehr als einer nicht diploiden Stammzellinie (Abb. 6). Bei einer weiteren Differenzierung des Kollektives wird deutlich, daß die Ploidie einen Einfluß auf das Überleben nur im Stadium III hat, im Stadium IV mit Streuung des Tumors außerhalb der Peritonealhöhle spielt der DNA-Gehalt keine Rolle mehr (Abb. 7).

In einer multivariaten Analyse unter Zuhilfenahme des Cox Regressionsmodelles haben wir überprüft inwieweit diese Variablen unabhängige prognostische Bedeutung besitzen. Es zeigte sich, daß das entscheidende Kriterium der postoperative Tumorrest ist, gefolgt vom Grading, der Ploidiestatus ist keine unabhängige prognostische Variable (Tabelle 1). Als Untergruppe mit etwas besserer Prognose lassen sich Patientinnen im Stadium III mit diploiden Tumoren festmachen.

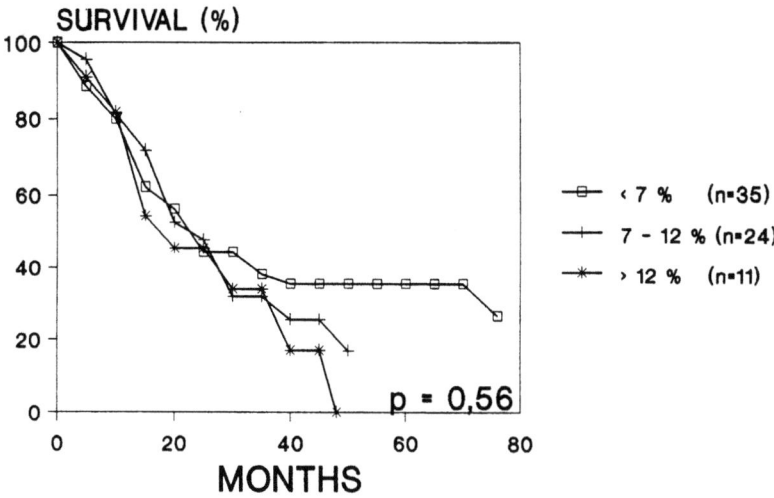

Abb. 8: SPF - Überlebenszeit; Stadium III+IV - diploide Tumoren

Tabelle 1: Multivariate analysis; stage III+IV

	Beta	Std. error	p
Resid. Tumor	1,32426	0,34631	0,0001
Grading	0,54959	0,27772	0,0478
Stage	0,15439	0,17350	0,3735
Ploidy	0,12338	0,17931	0,4914

Nun zur S-Phase als Maß der proliferativen Aktivität. Es fand sich kein Zusammenhang zwischen Ansprechen auf eine durchgeführte Chemotherapie und der S-Phase. In drei Gruppen mit niedriger, mittlerer und hoher proliferativer Aktivität unterteilt, wird deutlich, daß zwischen S-Phase und Überleben kein Zusammenhang besteht, obwohl nach 40 Monaten die Kurven divergierend verlaufen und in der Gruppe der Patienten mit niedriger S-Phase noch doppelt so viele leben wie in der mit hoher S-Phase (Abb. 8).

Es läßt sich festhalten, daß der nucleäre DNA-Gehalt mit dem Stadium, dem Alter, dem Grading, dem postoperativen Tumorrest sowie dem serösen Typ korreliert ist. Die zweifelsohne zwischen diesen Faktoren bestehenden Zusammenhänge bedürfen der weiteren Analyse. Als Untergruppe mit besserer Prognose lassen sich diploide Tumoren im Stadium III ausmachen. Die Ursache hierfür ist unklar. Eine mögliche Erklärung könnte ein primär multifocales Tumorwachstum in der Peritonealhöhle aufgrund des sogenannten »Müller'schen Potentials« der Zellen darstellen. Bei diesen Stadium III Fällen würde es sich also bei den in der Peritonealhöhle gefundenen Tumoranteilen nicht um Metastasen, sondern um zeitgleiches Entstehen mit den in den Ovarien entstandenen Tumorzellpopulationen im Sinne eines multifocalen Tumorwachstums handeln. Eine Untergruppe mit schlechter Prognose stellen multiploide Tumoren im Stadium III und IV dar. Die Ursache hierfür ist ebenfalls unbekannt. Es liegt hier offensichtlich eine weite zytogenetische Variabilität vor, was einerseits die Folge eines Zusammenbruches intratumoraler Regelkreise ist, andererseits ein therapeutisches Vorgehen wesentlich erschwert.

Die S-Phase als Maß der proliferativen Aktivität spielt weder beim Ansprechen des Tumors auf eine Chemotherapie noch hinsichtlich des Überlebens eine Rolle. Offensichtlich ist sie als Proliferationsmarker im Stadium III und IV ein zu einfaches Modell für die tumorbiologische Heterogenität dieser Tumoren. So werden zusätzliche Faktoren wie das Vorliegen einer primären Chemotherapieresistenz bzw. die sekundäre Entwicklung einer solchen nicht erfaßt.

Dennoch ist der zelluläre DNA-Gehalt ein objektiver, technisch einfach evaluierbarer und klinisch relevanter Parameter bei der Diagnostik und Therapie des Ovarialkarzinomes.

Literatur

1. Hedley D.W., Friedlander M.L., Taylor I.W., Rugg C.A., Musgrove E.A.: Method for analysis of cellular DNA content of paraffin-embedded pathological material using flowcytometry. J. Histochem. Cytochem. 31: 1333-1335, 1993

Steroid Rezeptoren beim Ovarialkarzinom: Die immunhistochemische Bestimmung birgt neue Perspektiven

F. Kommoss, J. Pfisterer, M. Thome, W. Sauerbrei, A. Pfleiderer

Abstract

Gewebsproben von 87 primären Ovarialkarzinomen des Stadiums FIGO III/IV wurden immunhistochemisch (IHC=Immunhistochemie) sowie biochemisch (DCC=Dextran-Coated Charcoal Methode) auf ihren Gehalt von Östrogenrezeptor (ER) und Progesteronrezeptoren (PR) untersucht. Während mittels DCC 62% der Tumoren ER sowie 66% PR positiv waren, konnte die IHC nur in 38% ER positive sowie in 31% PR positive maligne Tumorepithelien zeigen. Es bestand zudem nur eine niedrige Korrelation zwischen den semiquantitativen Scores der ER und PR IHC und den jeweiligen Ergebnissen der DCC Rezeptor Bestimmung. Benigne Steroidrezeptor positive Zellen des Tumorstromas bei andererseits gänzlich negativen Tumorepithelien könnten häufig beobachtete diskrepante Ergebnisse beider Methoden mit »falsch positivem« DCC Wert erklären. Die meisten Patientinnen wurden radikal operiert (n=76) und erhielten eine platinhaltige Chemotherapie (n=79). Während ER im vorliegenden Kollektiv keine signifikante prognostische Bedeutung hatte, hatten Patientinnen mit PR positiven Tumoren (IHC und DCC) bei univariater Analyse einen signifikanten Überlebensvorteil. Nach multivariater Analyse zeigte nur der postoperative Tumorrest eine eindeutige prognostische Signifikanz. In weiteren Studien sollte die biologische Bedeutung Steroidrezeptor positiver Stromazellen in Ovarialkarzinomen untersucht werden.

Einleitung

Mittels konventioneller biochemischer Methoden konnten in 62% aller Ovarialkarzinome ER sowie in 49% PR nachgewiesen werden [1]. Obwohl manche Autoren über eine prognostische Bedeutung des ER [2] oder PR [3,4,5,6] beim Ovarialkarzinom berichtet haben, wird dies noch immer kontrovers diskutiert, da andere Gruppen diese Ergebnisse nicht bestätigen konnten [7,8]. Die ER und PR DCC Analyse bestimmt den durchschnittlichen Rezeptorgehalt in Gewebshomogenisaten. Die IHC dahingegen ermöglicht eine exakte

Beschreibung der Steroidrezeptor positiven Gewebskomponente. Erste Studien mit dieser Methode haben gezeigt, daß möglicherweise deutlich weniger Ovarialkarzinome ER [9] oder PR [10] positiv sind als bislang angenommen. Es war daher unser Bestreben, den ER und PR Gehalt mittels IHC und DCC an einer Serie primärer fortgeschrittener Ovarialkarzinome zu bestimmen und die Ergebnisse auf ihre prognostische Bedeutung hin zu untersuchen.

Material und Methoden

Patienten, klinisches Vorgehen

87 Patientinnen mit einem primären, nicht vorbehandelten Ovarialkarzinom im FIGO Stadium III/IV wurden in die Studie aufgenommen. Das primäre Behandlungskonzept bestand in den meisten Fällen aus radikaler zytoreduktiver Operation (n=76) und aus minimal 2 Zyklen platinhaltiger Chemotherapie (n=79). Die second-line Therapie wurde individuell gehandhabt, häufig kamen mehrere Zyklen einer Vepesid® (Etoposid) Chemotherapie zum Einsatz. Zum Zeitpunkt der Auswertung waren 48 Patientinnen an ihrem Tumor verstorben.

Tumor Material

Tumorgewebe wurde anläßlich der Primäroperation an der Universitäts-Frauenklinik Freiburg gewonnen. Repräsentatives vitales Gewebe wurde rasch in flüssigem Stickstoff eingefroren und bei -70°C bis zur Weiterverarbeitung aufbewahrt. Unter 87 epithelialen Ovarialkarzinomen befanden sich 61 papillär seröse, 10 undifferenzierte solide, 9 endometrioide, 4 muzinöse und 3 klarzellige Tumore. Die Gewebsproben wurden in zwei gleiche Teile zur immunhistochemischen und biochemischen Rezeptoranalyse aufgeteilt.

ER und PR Immunhistochemie

Die IHC wurde gemäß des bereits publizierten Protokolls unter Anwendung käuflicher ER und PR Kits (Abott GmbH, Wiesbaden) am Gefrierschnitt durchgeführt [10]. Die mikroskopische Auswertung der Immunfärbungen erfolgte an einem Leitz Diaplan Mikroskop. Semiquantitative Immunoreaktive Scores (0-12) [11] wurden erstellt, zudem erfolgte eine Einstufung des Rezeptorverteilungsmusters. Typ-A Tumoren zeigen hierbei eine uniforme intensive Anfärbung sämtlicher epithelialer Tumorzellen, wohingegen Typ-B Tumoren sowohl gänzlich negative als auch stark positive Tumorepithelien enthalten. Typ-C Tumoren enthalten ein breites Spektrum von negativen über schwach positive bis zu stark positiven Tumorzellen [12]. Spezifische Immunpräzipitate in den Zellkernen benigner Stromazellen, welche in manchen Tumoren angetroffen wurden, blieben für die immunhistochemische Einstufung des Rezeptorstatus unberücksichtigt.

ER und PR DCC Analyse

Die biochemische Rezeptorbestimmung erfolgte gemäß des publizierten Protokolls [10]. Die Radioliganden 6,7-^{3}H Östradiol und 17α-methyl-^{3}H-Promegeston (NEN, Dreieich) kamen zum Einsatz. Der Schwellenwert für Rezeptorpositivität wurde bei einer Bindungskapazität von minimal 10 fmol/mg Gewebsprotein festgelegt.

Statistik

Spearman's rank Korrelationskoeffizienten wurden für die Analyse des Zusammenhangs zwischen Steroid Rezeptoren und den anderen prognostischen Faktoren berechnet. Die Überlebenszeiten wurden vom Zeitpunkt der Primäroperation bis zum Todestag oder zum Tag des letzten Patientenkontaktes berechnet. Überlebensraten wurden nach der Kaplan-Meier Methode geschätzt [13]. Univariate Effekte wurden mittels Log rank und Wilcoxon Test für zensierte Daten beurteilt [14]. Der Einfluß prognostischer Faktoren wurde multivariat nach dem Cox-Modell untersucht [15]. Sämtliche Berechnungen wurden auf dem Statistischen Analyse System (SAS) durchgeführt.

Tabelle 1: Patientenmerkmale, Prognostische Faktoren, Steroid Rezeptoren (n=87)

	n	%	ER positiv IHC	ER positiv DCC	PR positiv IHC	PR positiv DCC
Grad						
1	7	8	7	3	7	7
2&3	80	92	26	51	20	51
FIGO Stadium						
III	66	76	24	41	21	47
IV	21	24	9	13	6	11
Alter (Jahre)						
≤60	32	37	14	20	13	24
>60	55	63	19	34	14	34
Histologie						
serös	61	70	27	43	22	42
nicht serös	26	30	6	11	5	16
Tumorrest postp. (cm)						
≤0,05	19	22	10	12	11	16
>0,5	68	78	23	42	16	42

Ergebnisse

Prognostische Faktoren

Die Verteilung der prognostischen Faktoren Grad (2&3 vs. 1, Stadium (III vs. IV), Alter (>60 vs. ≤60 Jahre), Histologie (serös vs. nicht-serös) und postoperativer Tumorrest (>0,5cm vs. ≤0,5cm) sowie ihre Beziehung zum Steroidrezeptorstatus sind aus Tabelle 1 ersichtlich.

IHC

33 Tumore (38%) waren ER positiv, 27 Tumore (31%) waren PR positiv. 18 Karzinome (21%) waren ER+/PR+, 15 (17%) ER+/PR-, 9 (10%) ER-/PR+ und 45 (52%) waren ER-/PR-. 33/33 ER positiven Tumoren wiesen ein Typ-C Rezeptor Verteilungsmuster auf. 7/27 PR positiven Karzinomen zeigten ein Typ-B, die übrigen 20/27 Fälle ein Typ-C Verteilungsmuster. Es fanden sich keine Ovarialkarzinome mit einem Typ-A Rezeptor Verteilungsmuster.

DCC

54 Tumore (62%) waren ER positiv, 58 Tumore (66%) waren PR positiv. 42 Karzinome (48%) waren ER+/PR+. 12 (14%) ER+/PR-, 16 (18%) ER-/PR+ und 17 (20%) waren ER-/PR-.

IHC vs. DCC

Zwischen beiden Methoden bestand eine 64% (n=56) Übereinstimmung bei der Einstufung des ER und PR Status. Bei den meisten der 31 Tumore mit diskordanten Ergebnissen fand sich eine negative ER oder PR IHC bei positiven DCC Ergebnissen. (Tabellen 2 und 3). ER spezifische Immunpräzipitate in Zellkernen benigner Stromazellen ohne solche Immunfärbung von epithelialen Tumorzellkernen fanden sich in 5 Ovarialkarzinomen. 12 Tumore enthielten neben PR positiven Stromazellen ausschließlich PR negative Tumorepithelien (Abb. 1). Sämtliche der letztgenannten Karzinome waren in der DCC Analyse ER oder PR positiv gewesen. Die Regressionsanalyse zeigte eine mäßige Korrelation zwischen den quantitativen Ergebnissen der DCC Methode und den jeweiligen semiquantitativen immunoreaktiven Scores für ER und PR (Spearman's rank Korrelationskoeffizient 0,48 für ER, 0,56 für PR).

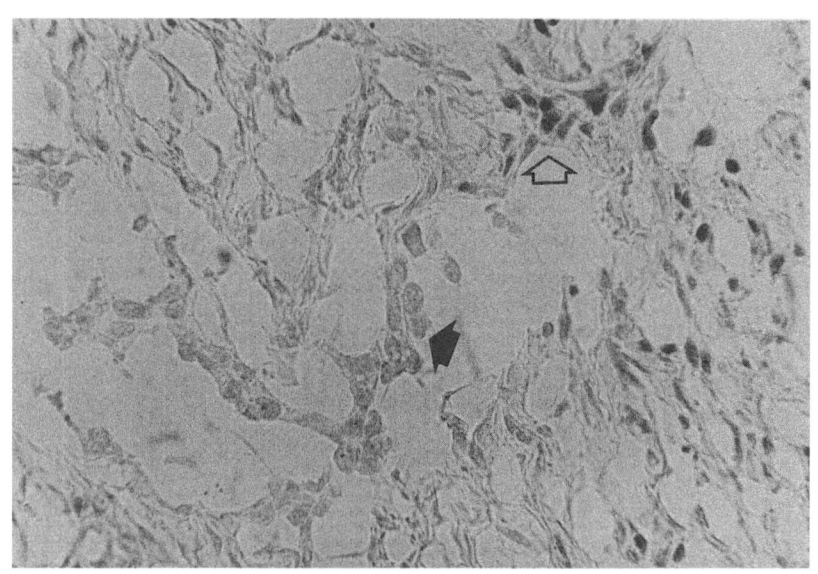

Abb. 1: Gering differenziertes papillär seröses Ovarialkarzinom, PR Immunhistochemie. Das Tumorepithel ist PR negativ (dunkler Pfeil), benigne spindelförmige Stromazellen zeigen PR spezifische Immunpräzipiate (heller Pfeil). PR IRS=0, PR DCC=125 fmol/mg Protein.

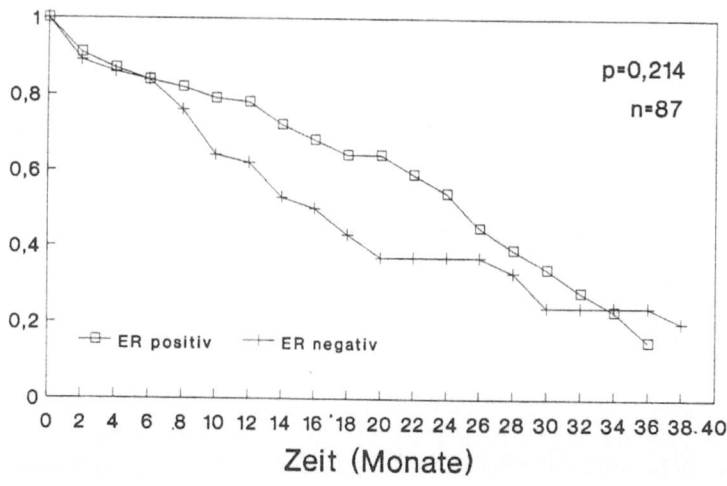

Abb. 2: Überleben bei Ovarialkarzinomen; ER, Immunhistochemie: ER (IHC) ist kein signifikanter prognostischer Faktor in einer Serie von 87 primären Ovarialkarzinomen im FIGO Stadium III/IV.

Tabelle 2: ER Status bei Ovarialkarzinomen; IHC vs. DCC, n=87

		DCC			
		neg.	pos.		
IHC	neg	28	26	54	
	pos	5	28	33	alle Typ C
		33	54	87	

Tabelle 3: PR Status bei Ovarialkarzinomen; IHC vs. DCC, n=87

		DCC			
		neg.	pos.		
IHC	neg	28	32	60	
	pos	1	26	27	Typ-B n=7 Typ-C n=20
		29	58	87	

Überleben

Trotz positiver Tendenz bei ER positiven Tumoren zeigte sich bei univariater Betrachtungsweise keine prognostische Signifikanz für ER IHC und DCC (Abb. 2 und 3). Bei PR positiven Fällen hingegen zeigte sich unabhängig von der Bestimmungsmethode ein signifikanter überlebensvorteil (DCC: log rank & Wilcoxon, IHC: Wilcoxon) (Abb. 4 und 5). In einem multivariaten Cox Modell [Parameter: PR (DCC), Tumor Histologie, Grade, Stage, Alter und postoperativer Tumorrest] zeigte lediglich der postoperative Tumorrest einen signifikanten prognostischen Effekt (Tabelle 4).

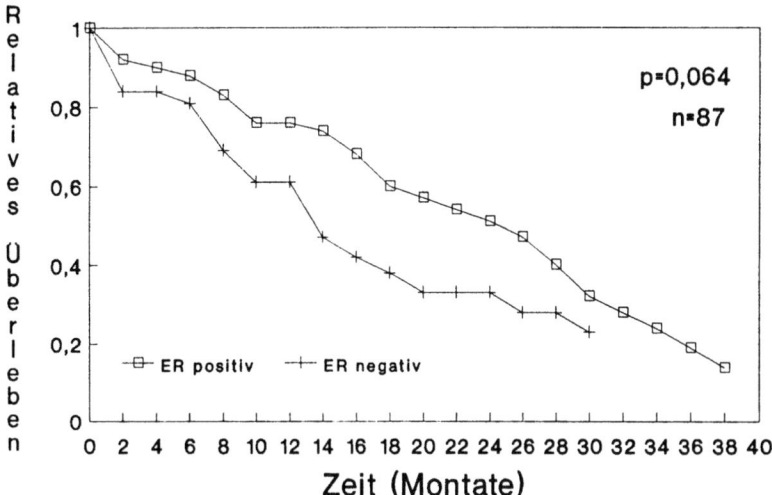

Abb. 3: Überleben bei Ovarialkarzinomen; ER, DCC: ER (DCC) ist kein signifikanter prognostischer Faktor in einer Serie von 87 primären Ovarialkarzinomen im FIGO Stadium III/IV.

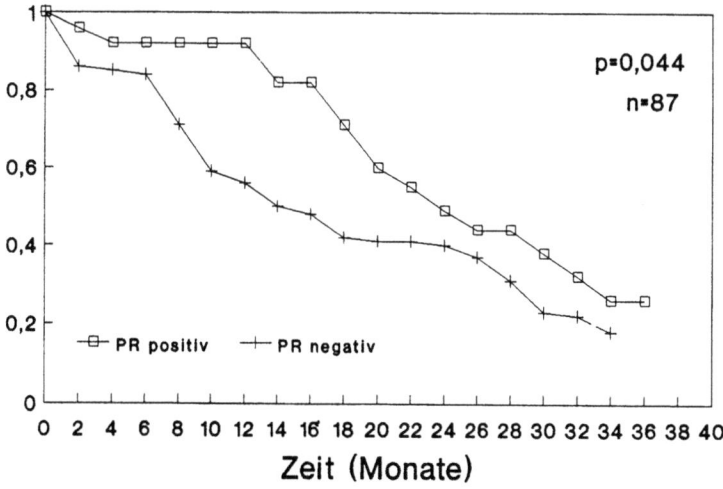

Abb. 4: Überleben bei Ovarialkarzinomen; PR, Immunhistochemie: PR (IHC) ist (univariat) ein signifikanter prognostischer Faktor in einer Serie von 87 primären Ovarialkarzinomen im FIGO Stadium III/IV.

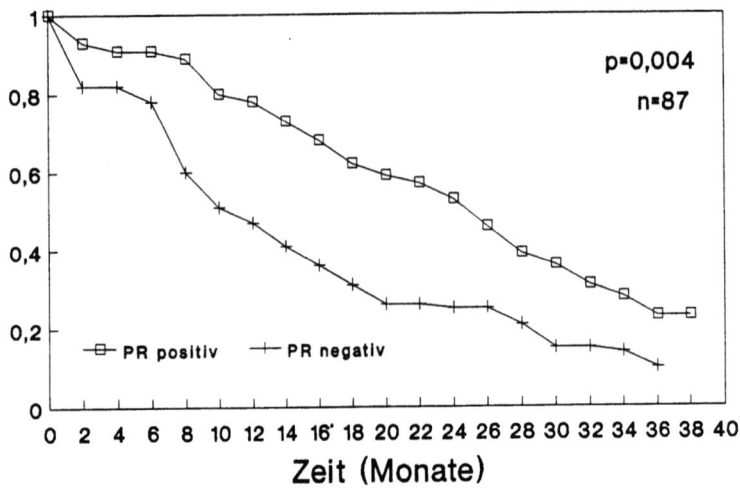

Abb. 5: Überleben bei Ovarialkarzinomen; PR, DCC: PR (DCC) ist (univariat) ein signifikanter prognostischer Faktor in einer Serie von 87 primären Ovarialkarzinomen im FIGO Stadium III/IV.

Tabelle 4: Multivariate (Cox) Regressions Analyse: Relative Risiken (R.R.) 95% Konfidenz Intervalle (95% K.I.), p-Werte (gemäß standardisierten Schätzwerten, »Wald-Test«)

Variable	R.R	95% K.I.	p
PR DCC (pos. vs. neg.)	0,60	0,33-1,09	0,098
Grade (2&3 vs. 1)	0,24	0,04-1,42	0,117
Stage (IV vs. III)	1,68	0,92-3,09	0,092
Alter (>60 vs. ≤60 Jahre)	1,80	0,85-3,82	0,122
Histologie (serös vs. nicht-s.)	1,39	0,72-2,70	0,326
Tumorrest (>0,5 vs. ≤0,5cm)	3,63	1,09-12,06	0,035

Diskussion

In dieser Untersuchung an 87 primären epithelialen Ovarialkarzinomen im Stadium III/IV wurde der Gehalt des Tumorgewebes an ER und PR mittels IHC und DCC Analyse bestimmt. Während der Anteil gemäß der DCC Methode ER oder PR positiver Tumoren (62% bzw. 66%) sehr ähnlich bzw. geringfügig höher war als in der Literatur beschrieben [1], war die Inzidenz von

Ovarialkarzinomen, welche immunhistochemisch ER oder PR positive maligne Epithelien enthielten, mit 38% bzw. 31% erstaunlich niedrig. Es bestand eine niedrige Korrelation zwischen den semiquantitativen immunoreaktiven Scores der IHC und den dazugehörigen DCC Zytosol Werten. Eine Abnahme der Rezeptorimmunogenität könnte im Laufe der Gewebsaufbewahrung und -verarbeitung aufgetreten sein und somit zu falsch negativen IHC Ergebnissen geführt haben. Ebenso könnte die bei Ovarialkarzinomen nicht ungewöhnliche Gewebsheterogenität [16] die differierenden Ergebnisse teilweise erklären. Es fiel allerdings auf, daß die meisten der Tumore mit diskordanten Ergebnissen immunhistochemisch Rezeptor negativ, jedoch positiv in der DCC Analyse waren. Das Vorkommen Rezeptor positiver benigner Stromazellen in ansonsten gänzlich negativen Tumoren erscheint uns daher eine noch einleuchtendere Erklärung für die offensichtliche Diskrepanz. Da über ähnlich »falsch positive« Ergebnisse der DCC Rezeptor Analyse auch bei Keimzelltumoren des Ovars [17], bei Borderline Tumoren des Ovars und bei Ovarialmetastasen [10] berichtet wurde, erscheint uns die IHC die geeignetere Methode der Steroidrezeptor Bestimmung bei Ovarialtumoren zu sein. Während der ER Status in unserer Serie keine signifikante prognostische Bedeutung aufwies, überlebten Patientinnen mit PR positiven Tumoren (IHC und DCC) signifikant länger. Allerdings war dieser Überlebensvorteil nach multivariater Analyse nicht mehr statistisch signifikant.

Unsere Ergebnisse stimmen mit Angaben in der Literatur überein [3,4,5]; Sevelda et al. fanden in einer Untersuchung einer großen Serie fortgeschrittener Ovarialkarzinome sogar eine unabhängige signifikante prognostische Bedeutung des PR (DCC) nach multivariater Analyse [6]. Obwohl bei der endokrinen Therapie vorbehandelter fortgeschrittener Tumoren über Response Raten von 9% (Tamoxifen [18]) und 15% (Gestagene [19], LHRH-Agonisten [20]) berichtet wurde, spielt diese Therapiemodalität bislang keine ernstzunehmende Rolle bei der Primärtherapie des Ovarialkarzinoms. Es ist bislang unklar, welche Komponente des Tumorgewebes das Ziel einer gelegentlich doch erfolgreichen endokrinen Therapie beim Ovarialkarzinom darstellt.

Wir konnten in dieser Studie zeigen, daß neben den Tumorepithelien (anders als bei Mammakarzinomen [12,21]) in Ovarialkarzinomen auch benigne Stromazellen ER und PR enthalten können. Eine steroidabhängige parakrine Interaktion zwischen beiden Gewebskomponenten erscheint somit vorstellbar. In zukünftigen Studien sollte die tumorbiologische Bedeutung Steroidrezeptor positiver Stromazellen in Ovarialkarzinomen untersucht werden.

Literatur

1. Rao B.R., Slotman B.J.: Endocrine factors in common epithelial ovarian cancer. Endocr. Rev. 12: 14-26, 1991
2. Bizzi A., Codegoni A.M., Landoni F., Marelli G., Marsoni S., Spina A.M., Torri W., Mangioni C.: Steroid receptors in epithelial ovarian carcinoma: relation to clinical parameters and survival, Cancer Res. 48: 6222-6226, 1988
3. Iversen O.E., Skaarland E., Utaaker E.: Steroid receptor content in human ovarian tumors: survival of patients with ovarian carcinoma related to steroid receptor content. Gynecol. Oncol. 23: 65-76, 1986
4. Slotman B.J., Kühnel R., Rao R.B., Dijhuizen G.H., De Graaff J., Stolk J.G.: Importance of steroid receptors and aromatase activity in the prognosis of ovarian cancer: high tumor progesterone receptor levels correlate with longer survival. Gynecol. Oncol. 33: 76-81, 1989
5. Harding M., Cowan S., Hole D., Cassidy L., Kitchener H., Davis J., Leake R.: Estrogen and progesterone receptors in ovarian cancer. Cancer 65: 486-491, 1990
6. Sevelda P., Denison U., Schemper M., Spona J., Vavra M., Salzer H.: Oestrogen and progesterone receptor content as a prognostic factor in advanced epithelial ovarian carcinoma, Br. J. Obstet. Gynaecol. 97: 706-712, 1990
7. Masood S., Heitmann J., Nuss R.C., Benrubi G.I.: Clinical correlation of hormone receptor status in epithelial ovarian cancer. Gynecol. Oncol. 34: 57-60, 1989
8. Anderl P., Fuith L.C., Daxenbichler G., Marth C., Dapunt O.: Correlation between steroid hormone receptors, histological and clinical parameters in ovarian carcinoma. Gynecol. Obstet. Invest. 25: 135-140, 1988
9. Isola J., Kallioniemi O.P., Korte J.M., Wahlströhm R., Aine R., Helle M., Helin H.: Steroid receptors and Ki-67 reactivity in ovarian cancer and in normal ovary: correlation with DNA flowcytometry, biochemical assay, and patient survival. J. Pathol. 162: 295-301, 1990
10. Kommoss F., Pfisterer J., Thome M., Geyer H., Sauerbrei W., Pfleiderer A.: Estrogen and progesterone receptors in ovarian neoplasms: discrepant results of immunohistochemical and biochemical results. Int. J. Gynecol. Cancer 1: 147-153, 1991
11. Remmele W., Stegner H.E.: Immunhistochemischer Nachweis von Östrogenrezeptoren (ER-ICA) in Mammakarzinomgewebe: Vorschlag zur einheitlichen Formulierung des Untersuchungsbefundes, Deutsches Ärzteblatt 83: 3362-3364, 1986
12. Kommoss F., Bibbo M., Colley M., Dytch H.E., Franklin W.A., Holt J.A., Wied G.L.: Distribution patterns and quantitation of hormone receptors in breast carcinoma by immunocytochemistry and image analysis. Part I: progesterone receptors. Analyt. Quant. Cytol. Histol. 11: 298-306, 1989
13. Kaplan E.L., Meier P.: Nonparametric estimation from incomplete observations. J. Am. Statist. Assoc. 53: 457-481, 1958
14. Kalbfleisch J.D., Prentice R.L.: The statistical analysis of failure time data. Wiley, New York, 1980

15. Cox D.R.: Regression models and life tables. J. Royal Statistical Society B 34: 187-220, 1972
16. Quinn M.A., Rome R.M., Cauchi M., Fortune D.W.: Steroid receptors and ovarian tumors: variation within primary tumors and between primary tumors and metastases. Gynecol. Oncol. 31: 424-429, 1988
17. Kommoss F., Franklin W.A., Talerman A.: Estrogen and progesterone receptors in Endodermal Sinus (Yolk sac) Tumor. Evaluation of immunocytochemical and biochemical methods. J. Reproductive Medicine 34: 943-945, 1989
18. Meerpohl H.G.: Palliative Hormontherapie beim Ovarialkarzinom. in: Aktuelle Onkologie 46: Antiöstrogene in Forschung und Klinik (Meerpohl H.G., Kaufmann M., Alt D., Pfleiderer A., Eds.), Zuckschwerdt Verlag München: 210-221, 1989
19. Slotman B.J., Rao B.R.: Ovarian cancer (review). Etiology, diagnosis, surgery, radiotherapy, chemotherapy, and endocrine therapy. Anticancer Res. 8: 417-434, 1988
20. Parmar H., Rustin G., Lightman S.L., Phillips R.H., Hanham I.W., Schally A.V.: Response to D-Trp-6-luteinizing hormone releasing (Decapeptyl) microcapsules in advanced ovarian cancer. Br. Med. J. 296: 1229, 1988
21. Colley M., Kommoss F., Bibbo M., Dytch H.E., Holt J.A., Wied G.L., Franklin W.A.: Assessment of hormone receptors in breast carcinoma by immunocytochemistry and image analysis. II. Estrogen Receptors. Analyt. Quant. Cytol. Histol. 11: 307-314, 1989

Klinische und prognostische Bedeutung tumorassoziierter Proteasen in der gynäkologischen Onkologie

W. Kuhn, F. Jänicke, O. Wilhelm, M. Schmitt, H. Graeff

Die Bösartigkeit solider Tumoren beinhaltet ihre Fähigkeit zur Invasion und Metastasierung. Neuere Ergebnisse der grundlagenorientierten und klinischen Forschung zeigen, daß die Tumorzelle selbst über ein großes Arsenal an Substanzen verfügt, um die Strukturen ihrer unmittelbaren Umgebung aufzubauen und auch wieder aufzulösen. Damit ist es ihr möglich, z.b. über den Abbau der extrazellulären Matrix und der Basalmembran, sich in das sie umgebende Gewebe auszubreiten und in Gefäße einzubrechen. In entsprechender Weise erfolgt durch verschleppte Tumorzellen bzw. Zellembolien nach Adhäsion im Gefäßbereich von Lunge, Leber, Knochen oder anderen Organen die Penetration der Gefäßwand und die Invasion des darunterliegenden Gewebes. Da die Struktur der zu durchdringenden Gewebe vorwiegend von Proteinen, Proteoglykanen und Kollagen gebildet wird, handelt es sich bei den Substanzen, die die Tumorzelle zur Invasion und Metastasierung benutzt, vorwiegend um Proteasen. In besonderer Weise sind es hierbei Faktoren der Blutgerinnung und der Fibrinolyse, die über den Auf- und Abbau einzelner Komponenten der Tumor-Matrix an diesen Prozessen direkt und über die Aktivierung anderer Proteasesysteme indirekt beteiligt sind.

Das Tumorstroma liefert auch Gefäßbindegewebe und somit die Voraussetzung für die anschließend einsetzende Kapillareinsprossung, die wiederum den Anschluß des Tumorgewebes an das Gefäßsystem des Wirtsorganismus ermöglicht. Gerade die Frage der Neovaskularisation ist für das Wachstum und die Ausbreitung solider Tumoren von wesentlicher Bedeutung, sie benötigen die Vaskularisation ihres Stromas zur Anlieferung von Energieträgern und Sauerstoff, sowie zum Abtransport von Stoffwechselprodukten. Im folgenden sollen Aspekte der tumorassoziierten Proteolyse dargestellt werden, deren klinische Bedeutung sich schon jetzt abzeichnet.

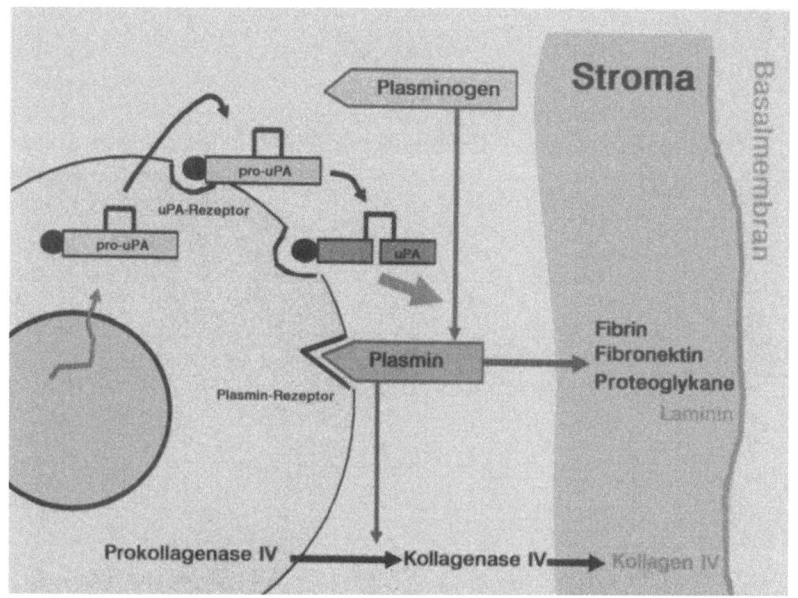

Abb. 1: Vereinfachte Darstellung der proteolytischen Vorgänge an der Tumorzelloberfläche und im Tumorstroma uPA = Plasminogenaktivator vom Urokinasetyp, pro-uPA = inaktive Vorstufe des Plasminogenaktivators vom Urokinasetyp.

Matrixabbau beim Ovarialkarzinom

Bisher experimentell und an Zellkulturen erhobene Befunde über den Abbau einer provisorischen »Fibrin-Fibronektin-Gelmatrix« konnten am Beispiel des Ovarialkarzinoms durch kliniknahe Beobachtungen unterstützt und für die Verhältnisse beim Menschen belegt werden [1-5]. Über die Analyse von Tumorstromafragmenten konnte gezeigt werden, daß die Protease Plasmin den Abbau von Fibrin und Fibronektin bewirkt. Erst durch Untersuchungen am Substrat Fibrin mit der Charakterisierung der submolekularen Struktur quervernetzter löslicher Fibrinderivate und durch die Aminosäuresequenzanalyse der Untereinheiten (Peptidketten) von Fibrinabbauprodukten aus Ovarialkarzinomaszites konnte die allgemeine Annahme belegt werden, daß Plasmin die essentielle Protease ist, die den Abbau des Stromaanteils Fibrin bewirkt. Offensichtlich spielt die von Entzündungszellen gebildete Elastase beim Abbau des Fibrins im Tumorstroma keine wesentliche Rolle. Im Gegensatz zu den hohen Elastase-Spiegeln im entzündlichen Aszites ist Elastase im malignen Aszites nicht nachweisbar.

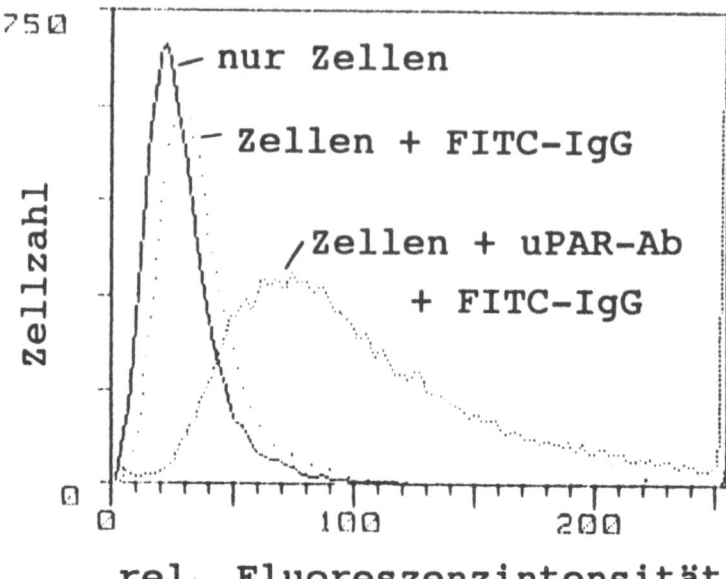

Abb. 2: Nachweis von upA-Rezeptoren auf Ovarialkarzinomzellen mittels Durchflußzytometrie. Die Zellinie OC-6 wurde aus einem primären Ovarialkarzinom etabliert (Möbus und Kreienberg, Universitätsfrauenklinik Mainz). OC-6 besitzt Rezeptoren für den Urokinase-Typ-Plasminogen Aktivator (uPA). uPA-Rezeptoren können auf der Zelloberfläche von OC-6 mittels Durchflußzytometrie nach Reaktion mit dem monoklonalen Antikörper 3936 (American Diagnostica, Greenwich, USA) nachgewiesen werden. Diese Technik kann zum Nachweis von uPA-Rezeptoren auf Zellen herangezogen werden, welche aus Tumorgeweben oder Aszitesflüssigkeiten gewonnen wurden.

Das Ausmaß der Tumorerkrankung beim Ovarialkarzinom korreliert mit dem Nachweis von Fibrin im Tumor und den Fibrinabbauproduktspiegeln im Aszites und im Blut. Über ROC-Diagramme, die unter Berücksichtigung von Sensitivität und Spezifität die Qualitäten verschiedener Tumormarker abschätzen lassen, wurde deutlich, daß der Nachweis von D-Dimer im Plasma der Bestimmung von CA-125 in der Wertigkeit als Tumormarker entsprach. Es soll damit nicht abgeleitet werden, CA-125, einen verläßlichen und allgemein eingeführten Tumormarker, durch D-Dimer zu ersetzen. Es kann jedoch aus diesen Beobachtungen über die Markerfunktion bestimmter im Plasma nachweisbarer Substanzen auf die tumorbiologische Bedeutung der hierdurch reflektierten Vorgänge geschlossen werden. Plasmin wird in der Umgebung von Tumorzellen aus dem enzymatisch inaktiven Plasmaprotein Plasminogen durch Einwirkung des Plasminogenaktivators Urokinase (uPA) gebildet. Zellen von Ovarial-, Zervix-, Endometrium- und Mamma-Karzinomen synthetisieren und sezernieren uPA als ein enzymatisch inaktives und einkettiges Proenzym (pro-Urokinase), das über den aminoterminalen Bereich des Moleküls auf spezifische Rezeptoren (uPA-Rezeptoren, uPAR) auf der Tumorzelloberfläche gebunden wird (Abb. 1). Neuere Untersuchungen zeigen, daß pro-Urokinase nicht nur durch Spuren von Plasmin, sondern auch durch die ebenfalls von der Tumorzelle gebildete Protease Kathepsin B [6] in die enzymatisch aktive Form (uPA) überführt wird. Rezeptorgebundener uPA (Abb. 2) überführt Plasminogen in Plasmin, dieses bindet dann in Nachbarschaft der uPA-Rezeptoren an Plasminrezeptoren auf der Tumorzelloberfläche. Während rezeptorgebundene Urokinase dem spezifischen Inhibitor Plasminogenaktivatorinhibitor 1 (PAI-1) zugänglich ist und hierdurch auch eine Limitierung der Urokinasewirkung erfolgen kann, ist rezeptorgebundenes Plasmin durch seine Inhibitoren nicht mehr hemmbar. Es entsteht ein rezeptorvermitteltes Proteasesystem auf der Tumorzelloberfläche, das über die Internalisation des Urokinase-PAI-1-Komplexes auch die Polarisierung der proteolytischen Aktivität auf der Zelloberfläche ermöglicht [7]. So kann die gerichtete Invasion von Tumorzellen in das umgebende Gewebe stattfinden.

uPA und PAI-1 als Prognosefaktoren beim Mammakarzinom

Nach Entwicklung eines Tests zur Messung des Gehalts von uPA-Antigen (ELISA-Technik) im Tumorgewebeextrakt konnte beim Mamma-Karzinom nachgewiesen werden, daß bei Patientinnen mit einem erhöhten uPA-Gehalt im Tumorgewebe schon nach einer mittleren Nachbeobachtungszeit von 12,5 Monaten signifikant gehäuft Rezidive auftraten [8]. Bestätigt wurde die überlegene prognostische Bedeutung des Urokinase-Antigennachweises gegenüber dem Nachweis der Urokinase-Aktivität von Duffy et al. [9]. Im weiteren konnte nach einer längeren Nachbeobachtungszeit von 25 Monaten gezeigt werden, daß in der Multivarianzanalyse Urokinase nicht nur bezogen auf das rezidivfreie Überleben, sondern auch in Bezug auf das Gesamtüberleben ein deutlich stärkerer Prognosefaktor ist als Hormonrezeptorstatus und Lymphkotenbefall [10]. Ähnliches gilt für den Inhibitor von uPA, PAI-1, der in hohen Konzentrationen im Mammakarzinomgewebe nachweisbar ist. Patientinnen mit hohen PAI-1-Spiegeln im Mammakarzinom haben eine signifikant höhere Rezidivrate und eine kürzere Gesamtüberlebenswahrscheinlichkeit als Patientinnen mit niederen PAI-1-Spiegeln. In der Multivarianzanalyse wird deutlich, daß der PAI-1-Gehalt eine prognostische Abschätzung erlaubt, die unabhängig

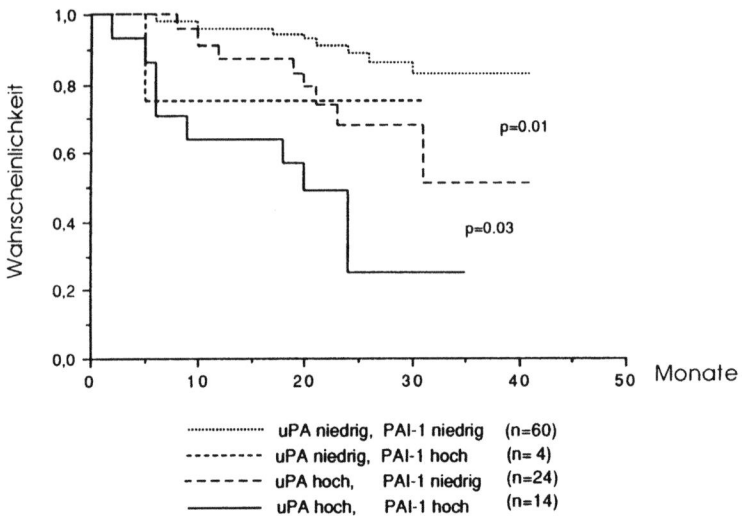

Abb. 3: Rezidivfreies Überleben bei Patientinnen mit primärem Mammakarzinom in Abhängigkeit vom uPA- und PAI-1-Gehalt im Tumorgewebe [nach 10].

vom uPA-Gehalt ist. Die Kombination der beiden Prognosefaktoren uPA und PAI-1 läßt Patientinnen mit einem hohen oder niederen Risiko für ein Rezidiv unabhängig von den klassischen Risikofaktoren (Lymphknotenstatus, Hormonrezeptorstatus) erkennen (Abb. 3).

uPA als Prognosefaktor beim Ovarialkarzinom

Neben dem Nachweis von D Dimer im Plasma und im malignen Aszites und dem Nachweis von Fibrin im Tumorgewebe ist es möglich, auch uPA in Ovarialkarzinomen nachzuweisen. In eigenen, noch nicht veröffentlichten Beobachtungen konnte gezeigt werden, daß in Ovarialkarzinomen uPA, PAI-1 und Kathepsin D in signifikant höheren Konzentrationen nachweisbar sind als in Gewebsproben aus gutartigem Ovarialgewebe. Im weiteren konnte nachgewiesen werden, daß durch die Messung des uPA-Gehaltes im Ovarialkarzinom eine Aussage über die Überlebenswahrscheinlichkeit der Patientinnen gemacht werden kann. So ist deutlich geworden, daß die Patientinnen, die im Rahmen der Primäroperation tumorfrei operiert werden konnten mit einem niedrigen uPA-Gehalt im Tumorgewebe eine signifikant längere mediane Überlebenszeit aufwiesen als die tumorfrei operierten Patientinnen mit hohem uPA-Gehalt im Tumorgewebe. Trotz dieser statistisch signifikanten Ergebnisse kann noch keine endgültige Aussage über die Wertigkeit des Prognosefaktors uPA im Vergleich zu den bisher etablierten Prognosekriterien gemacht werden, da aufgrund der relativ kleinen Fallzahl (n=15) eine Multivarianzanalyse für die einzelnen Prognosekriterien noch nicht machbar ist. Die bisher verwandten Prognosekriterien (Alter, Aszitesmenge, Grading, Tumorrest und andere) werden weiterhin ihre Gültigkeit behalten. Hierbei konnte in eigenen Beobachtungen gezeigt werden, daß der postoperative Tumorrest sowohl bei der Primär- als auch bei der Rezidivoperation bei multivariater Analyse den härtesten Prognoseparameter darstellt [11,12]. Zukünftig ist es jedoch durchaus denkbar, daß sich uPA als neuer Prognoseparameter etabliert, mit dem nicht nur eine Aussage über die Überlebenswahrscheinlichkeit der Patientinnen möglich ist, sondern der auch Einfluß auf die Auswahl postoperativer, adjuvanter Therapieformen hat.

Üblicherweise wird postoperativ eine platinhaltige, adjuvante Chemotherapie verabreicht. Diese ist integraler Bestandteil der Primärbehandlung der Patientinnen mit Ovarialkarzinom. Die Therapieplanung für Patientinnen mit LMP (Low Malignant Potential)-Karzinomen muß jedoch individualisierter gestaltet werden, da diese Karzinome aufgrund fehlender Stromainvasion üblicherweise eine deutlich bessere Prognose aufweisen als die invasiven Karzinome [13]. Bei diesen Karzinomen wird daher ein eingeschränktes radikales operatives Vorgehen diskutiert, zusätzlich scheint eine routinemäßige, postoperative adjuvante Chemotherapie in den meisten Fällen nicht indiziert zu sein. Auf der anderen Seite konnte gezeigt werden, daß bei über 30% der Patientinnen mit Low Malignant Potential Karzinomen peritoneale Metastasen nachweisbar sind und daß über 30% dieser Patientinnen an ihrer Tumorerkrankung versterben trotz fehlender Stromainvasion des Primärtumors [14].

Die Notwendigkeit, anhand von spezifischen Prognosefaktoren ein Risikokollektiv zu definieren, das dann von der adjuvanten Chemotherapie profitieren würde, wird somit anhand der obigen Zahlen deutlich.

Neben den Kriterien für Zellproliferation (S-Phase, Ploidie, DNA-Gehalt u.a.) zeichnet sich hier zusätzlich uPA als neuer Prognosefaktor ab.

Am Beispiel des Mammkarzinoms und des Ovarialkarzinoms ist deutlich geworden, daß die Erkenntnisse, die man über die tumorassoziierte Fibrinolyse gewonnen hat und die bei der Analyse von Krankheitsverläufen angewandt worden sind, zukünftig Einfluß auf therapeutische Entscheidungen haben können.

Darüber hinaus sind jedoch biologische Therapieformen denkbar, z.B. über die Hemmung der Urokinasesynthese oder über die Beeinflussung der Interaktion zwischen Urokinase und Urokinaserezeptor, um der Tumorausdehnung entgegenwirken zu können [15]. Einschränkend für die meisten der an der Tumorbiologie orientierten therapeutischen Ansätze gilt jedoch, daß es sich bei den Mechanismen, die die Tumorzelle z.B. durch Verwendung von Proteasen zur Invasion und Metastasierung benutzt, nicht um tumorzellspezifische pathophysiologische Prinzipien handelt, sondern um Mechanismen, die auch physiologischerweise von den Zellen des Organismus in Zusammenhang mit Regeneration, Wundheilung, Fortpflanzung u.a. benutzt werden. Es sind lediglich quantitative und lokale Aspekte, die physiologische Funktionen von der Tumorzellpathophysiologie trennen. Es bedarf daher sicherlich noch umfangreicher, zunächst experimenteller Forschungsarbeit, bis diese biologischen Therapieformen klinisch einsetzbar sind.

Literatur

1. Graeff H., Hafter R.: Clinical aspects of fibrinolysis. In: Bloom L., Thomas D.P. (eds): Haemostasis and Thrombosis. Edinburgh: Churchill Livingstone: 245-254, 1987
2. Hafter R., Klaubert W., Gollwitzer R., von Hugo R., Graeff H.: Crosslinked fibrin derivates and fibronectin in ascites fluid from patients with ovarian cancer compared to ascitic fluid in liver cirrhosis. Thromb. Res. 35: 53-64, 1984
3. Röbl M., Jürgensmeyer K., Hafter R., Schröck R., Wilhelm O., Babic R., Graeff H.: Relation of fibrin and tumor-associated antigens to the spread of ovarian cancer. Fibrinolysis 1. 1: 143-148, 1987
4. Wilhelm O., Hafter R., Coppenrath E., Pflanz M.A., Schmitt M., Babic R., Linke R., Gössner W., Graeff H.: Fibrin-fibronectin compounds in human ovarian tumor ascites and their possible relation to the tumor stroma. Cancer. Res. 48: 3507-3514, 1988
5. Wilhelm O., Hafter R., Henschen A., Schmitt M., Graeff H.: Role of plasmin in the degradation of the stroma-derived fibrin in human ovarian carcinoma. Blood 75: 1673-1678, 1990
6. Kobayashi H., Schmitt M., Goretzki L., Chucholowski N., Calvete J., Kramer M., Günzler W.A., Jänicke F., Graeff H.: Cathepsin B efficiently activates the soluble and the tumor cell receptor-bound form of the proenzyme urokinase-type plasminogen activator (pro-uPA). J. Biol. Chem. 266: 5147-5152, 1991

7. Cubellis M.V., Wun T., Blasi F.: Receptor-mediated internalization and degradation of urokinase is caused by its specific inhibitor PAI-1. EMBO J. 9: 1079-1085, 1990
8. Jänicke F., Schmitt M., Hafter R., Hollrieder A., Babic R., Ulm K., Gössner W., Graeff H.: Urokinase-type plasminogen activator (u-PA) antigen is a predictor of early relapse in breast cancer. Fibrinolysis 4: 69-78, 1990
9. Duffy M.J., Reilley D., O'Sullivan C., O'Higgins N., Fennelly J.J.: Urokinase plasminogen activator and prognosis in breast cancer. Lancet 8681: 108, 1990
10. Jänicke F., Schmitt M., Graeff H.: Clinical relevance of the urokinase-type and tissue-type plasminogen activators and of their type 1 inhibitor in breast cancer. Semin. Thromb. Hemost 17: 303-312, 1991
11. Jänicke F., Hölscher M., Kuhn W., v. Hugo R., Pache L., Siewert J.R., Graeff H.: Radical surgery improves survival in recurrent ovarian cancer. Cancer 1992 (in press)
12. Griffith C.T., Parker L.M., Fuller A.F. Jr.: Role of cytoreductive surgical treatment in the management of advanced ovarian cancer. Cancer Treat. Rep. 63: 235-240, 1979
13. Bostwick D.G., Tazelaar H.D., Ballon S.C., Hendrickson M.R., Kempson R.L.: Ovarian epithelial tumors of borderline malignancy. Cancer 58: 2052-2065, 1986
14. Bell D.A., Weinstock M.A., Scully R.E.: Peritoneal implants of ovarian serous borderline tumors. Histologic features and prognosis. Cancer 62: 2212-2222, 1988
15. Graeff H., Jänicke F., Schmitt M.: Klinische und prognostische Bedeutung tumorassoziierter Proteasen in der gynäkologischen Onkologie. Gebh. u. Frauenh. 51: 90-99, 1991

III. Screening, Staging, Imaging

Screening for Ovarian Cancer

S. Campbell, T. Bourne

Abstract

As a profession we devote a huge amount of time and money to the early detection and investigation of cervical and endometrial carcinoma. If one considers the fact that more women die each year from ovarian cancer than from cancer of the uterus and cervix combined, the failure to investigate methods to detect ovarian cancer at an early stage is puzzling. The relative lack of information regarding the natural history of ovarian cancer has hindered workers in this field. The result is that the vital question of whether screening for and thus early detection and treatment of ovarian cancer actually reduces mortality from the disease has yet to be answered. A randomised controlled clinical trial is needed to test this hypothesis. We believe that an ultrasound based screening test now exists with sufficient sensitivity and specificity to be utilised in the context of such a clinical trial. This article will set out the arguments for this proposal.

Introduction

5000 women develop ovarian cancer in England and Wales each year of whom about 4300 will die from their disease [1]. It is unusual for the disease to be symptomatic in its earliest stages, and as a result over 60% of women with this cancer present at a late surgical stage [2]. This factor is thought to contribute significantly to the overall five year survival rate which is less than 30%. The five year survival rate may be over 90% for well differentiated tumours confined to within the capsule of the ovaries (surgical stages Ia and Ib) [3]. Once the cancer has spread beyond the ovary the survival rate drops to 13% and 4% for stage III and stage IV disease respectively [4]. These data reflect the relative lack of progress towards effective treatments for this disease, and has led to attempts being made to develop screening procedures for the early stages of this cancer in asymptomatic women. Ideally screening would be directed towards detecting the disease at a premalignant phase, however no such stage has been described to date, and so the aim is to detect early invasive disease within the ovary. The issue of ovarian cancer screening has been reviewed [5].

Screening

Natural History of the disease

The World Health Organisation (WHO) has set out criteria that should be satisfied by a disease before screening is implemented [6]. Prominent amongst these is that the natural history of the disease in question must be understood. It is clear that for ovarian cancer this is not the case. It is becoming apparent that surgical stage does not give a sufficiently accurate indication of outcome. That ovarian cancers always progress through each surgical stage is not certain. The possibility that stage III disease may represent multifocal lesions originating from a primed peritoneum must be considered.

End points

Factors such as the ploidy status, nuclear morphometry, and the reaction of individual tumours to biological response modifiers (BRM's) are receiving increasing attention. The endpoints of screening studies are therefore changing. However for the present time it is not unreasonable to have the detection of early stage tumours as the aim of most studies. For our own purposes we define early ovarian cancer as being the stage of the disease that can be completely removed by surgery, ie the tumour is confined to within the capsule of the ovary with no evidence of metastases.

Lead and length time bias

The concepts of lead and length time bias must also be understood. That the earlier diagnosis of a cancer must lead to a reduction in mortality from the disease is an attractive but flawed argument. Earlier diagnosis may mean that whilst the time from diagnosis to death from the disease is longer, the chronological date of death remains unchanged (lead time bias). Similarly screening may tend to detect relatively indolent tumours that would have an inherently better prognosis whether they are picked up at screening or not (length time bias) [7]. A randomised controlled study is needed to answer these questions, this would involve several centres to include enough women to demonstrate a reduction in mortality.

Possible tests to be used in such a trial include bimanual pelvic examination, however although this is still an intrinsic part of any gynaecological examination it is relatively insensitive for the detection of the relatively small ovarian lesions thought to be associated with early carcinoma. This paper will therefore address the possible roles of the measurement of tumor related antigens in peripheral blood, and the use of pelvic ultrasonography.

Serum Tumour Associated Antigens

Since the development of techniques for the production of monoclonal antibodies, many antigens expressed by tumours have been identified. Several antibodies have been shown to bind to antigens expressed by epithelial malignancies [8], however as yet a tissue specific marker has not been identified.

CA 125: The first to be reported and most clinically useful of these markers has been CA 125. OC 125, the antibody that defines CA 125, binds to over 70% of non-mucinous epithelial ovarian cancers. However this fails to consider the limited expression of the antigen that occurs at early stages of the disease. The antigen is not specific for ovarian cancer, and the level of serum CA 125 may be raised in benign conditions such as endometriosis or during menstruation and pregnancy. The expression of this antigen has been reviewed extensively [9]. There is little doubt that CA 125 offers a useful marker of disease activity when following up patients after treatment for ovarian cancer. However the available data do not suggest that the measurement of CA 125 alone offers a viable screening test for this disease. A serum concentration of above 30 U/ml has generally been used as a cutoff to define raised levels in women from the general population. Data generated from the JANUS serum bank suggests that for a cutoff level of 35 U/ml the specificity of the test would be 95,4% and the corresponding sensitivity for stage I cancers presenting during the subsequent 18 months < 35% [10].

The use of multiple markers: Several workers have now assessed the efficacy of measuring multiple markers in an attempt to improve overall test performance [8]. In general this approach leads to increased sensitivity if a positive result is defined as a rise in the serum concentration of any one of the markers; however this also produces a substantial reduction in specificity. Defining a positive result on the basis of a simultaneous rise in all markers tends to enhance specificity at the expense of sensitivity.

The future: The main problem with the measurement of serum tumour markers is that all those currently available appear to lack sufficient sensitivity for use as a first stage screening test. The false positive rate is unlikely to present a practical problem, as this can be effectively reduced either by the use of pelvic ultrasonography [11] or serial measurements of CA 125 [12] as second stage tests. Perhaps the best approach to aim for would the development of a dipstick that could be used to detect antigenic fragments in urine. If a panel of markers could be incorporated into such as strip, a positive result could be defined by a rise in any of the single markers. The resulting high false positive rate could then be reduced by the use of pelvic ultrasonography as a second stage test. Those women with a positive urine dipstick, and a lesion seen on ultrasound could be referred for surgery. In this way the number of women going forward to an ultrasound based programme could be reduced.

Pelvic Ultrasonography

Transabdominal Ultrasonography
The first data to suggest that ultrasonography may be used to screen asymptomatic women for early ovarian caner was reported by Campbell et al. in 1982 [13] when he showed that it was possible to accurately record the morphology and volume of postmenopausal ovaries. In a subsequent trial the technique was used to screen 5479 self-referred asymptomatic women on three separate occasions [14]. A positive screen result was based on the finding of persistent abnormal ovarian morphology demonstrated on ultrasound with histological examination of removed tissues as the endpoint of the study. Five stage I primary ovarian cancers were detected, two at screen one and three at screen two. Within the limitations of the trial design the sensitivity was 100% and the specifitcity over three screenings was 97,7%. The odds of finding any ovarian tumour amongst women with a positive test result were 1:2, whilst for primary ovarian cancer the odds were 1:67. By reanalysing the data it was found that if a defined volume change was required to have occurred on repeat scan (a reduction in volume of less than one third) as well as abnormal morphology being present, the specificity could be improved. Using these criteria the odds of finding a primary cancer at surgery were reduced to 1:50 [15]. The problem with transabdominal ultrasonography is that the operator is unable to distinguish between benign and malignant cystic lesions on the basis of their appearance. Five malignant lesions (three primary and two metastatic tumours) in the series of Campbell et al [14] had a unilocular simple cystic structure. Similarly Luxman et al. [16] reported that 2 of 33 patients (6%) with simple cysts less than 5,0 cm as assessed by transabdominal ultrasonography had malignant ovarian tumours.

Performing fifty operations on women with ovarian cystic lesions to find one primary ovarian cancer may seem unacceptable, however the implications do deserve debate. Such a policy may be reasonable if a proportion of the benign lesions were to become malignant at a later date, or cause other mechanical problems. Thus the removal of these benign growths may lead to a reduction in the number of incident cases of carcinoma in the population. Furthermore recent advances in pelviscopic surgery may significantly alter the cost of a false positive test result [17]. However this hypothesis regarding the natural history of ovarian cancer is unsubstantiated, and so for the moment we must address the issue of improving test performance if a viable screening strategy is to be envisaged.

Transvaginal Ultrasonography
The practical use of this technique has been described in detail [18,19]. The transducer is placed closer to the area of interest, less of the ultrasound is absorbed, and so higher frequencies can be used. This leads to an improvement in the resolution of the images obtained. A further major practical advantage is that a full bladder is not required for the procedure to be performed. Ovarian volume and morphology assessed by transvaginal ultrasonography has been shown to correlate closely with the findings at surgery [20].

Preliminary data have already been published using this method to screen for primary ovarian carcinoma in an asymptomatic population [21]. In this study of the 9,2% of premenopausal women who had an ovarian lesion detected at initial scan only 3,8% remained by the time a repeat scan was performed 3 to 6 weeks later. The careful reassessment of a cyst found at screening is vital if a high false positive rate secondary to physiological lesions is to be avoided. No interval cancers have been detected at one year follow up of these women. In another study using this technique [22] 3 cases of stage I primary ovarian cancer have been detected in a cohort of 776 women with a family history of ovarian carcinoma. Again no interval cancers have been detected on follow up.

These preliminary data suggest that transvaginal ultrasonography provides a sensitive test for the early stages of ovarian cancer. The real issue is whether this probable high detection rate can be maintained whilst trying to achieve a reduction in the false positive rate of the screening procedure.

Improving the odds ratio of finding a cancer in patients referred for surgery
Addressing high risk groups: For any diagnostic test, the positive predictive value of a positive result is improved by directing it towards a group at increased risk of developing the disease in question. This is simply a reflection

Table 1: Screening for familial ovarian carcinoma. (Kings College Hospital Ovarian Scanninng clinic 1992). The prevalence of persistent ovarian masses in two populations of self-referred, asymptomatic women attending ultrasound based screening programmes.

	Study group		
Ovarian mass	General population Rate/1000 women	Cancer families Rate/1000 women	Rate ratio
Malignant epithelial	0,3	1,9	7,0
Benign epithelial	6,6	10,3	1,6
Sex cord stromal/germ cell	1,3	2,6	2,0
Tumour-like	6,3	20,8	3,3
Simple cysts	2,7	6,5	2,4
Follicular cysts	1,9	3,2	1,7
Corpus luteum cysts	0,7	7,1	10,1

of the increased amount of disease in the study population. A positive family history has been recognised as being an important risk factor for ovarian carcinoma [23]. We have studied 1110 women who have had at least one close relative develop the disease. The preliminary data have been published [22]. All the women have had both a transvaginal and transabdominal scan carried out. Four primary ovarian cancers have been detected, all at stage Ia. Both the prevalence of the disease and the predictive value of a positive test result are significantly higher than our previous population based trial [14] (table 1). Because of the increased disease prevalence the odds against finding a cancer amongst women with a positive screening test have been reduced to 1:14. When women are at such high risk further second stage tests may not be required. By examining women at increased risk of ovarian cancer the overall test performance has been enhanced. The current interest in the recognition of a genetic marker of disease risk is therefore of importance in selecting those women in whom screening is most likely to be worthwhile. The CRC genetics unit at Cambridge is currently running a trial under the auspices of the UKCCR to try and identify women with such dominant inheritance patterns so as to isolate the putative oncogene — clinicians who identify families falling into such groups should contact the unit for further details.

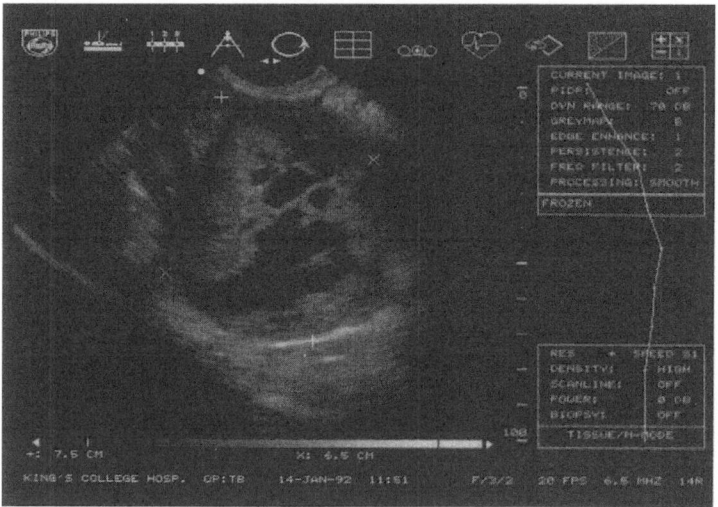

Fig. 1: An irregular lesion within a relatively small ovary. The papillary projections into the cyst are a highly suspicious feature.

The use of second stage tests — morphology scores and transvaginal colour Doppler Ultrasonography:
Previous studies using transabdominal ultrasonography have suggested that this technique cannot be used to discriminate between benign and malignant cystic lesions [14,24]. Greater success may be achieved by the use of high resolution transvaginal ultrasonography. There is a general view that a simple unilocular cystic lesion with no solid areas, a regular outline and anechoic contents, is highly unlikely to harbour a malignancy. In an attempt to quantitate this impression morphology scoring systems have been developed [25]. The problem in extrapolating this to the situation with screening is that little information is available regarding the structure of very early stage I lesions. Fig. 1 and 2 illustrate the morphological appearances of a benign lesion and an early carcinoma, note the solid papillary projection and irregular outline of the malignant lesion. What is clear however is that a simple unilocular cystic lesion in a postmenopausal women is not necessarily abnormal, and that if such a cyst is present it may regress. By carefully reassessing morphological abnormalities found on ultrasound a number of false positive test results can be avoided.

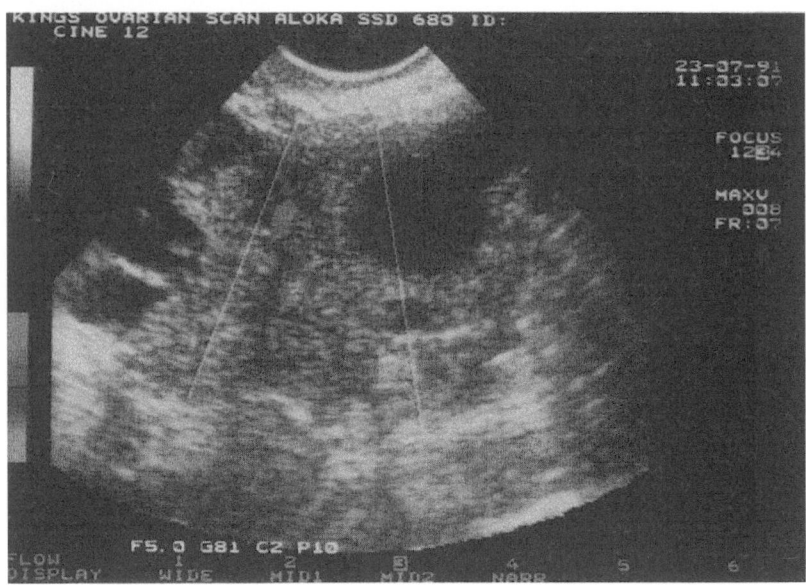

Fig. 2: (a) Presumed neovascularisation within a stage III primary ovarian carcinoma, (b) demonstrates the flow velocity waveform obtained from the same lesion - the presence of flow in the diastolic phase of the cardiac cycle implies low vascular impedance and is characteristic of carcinoma.

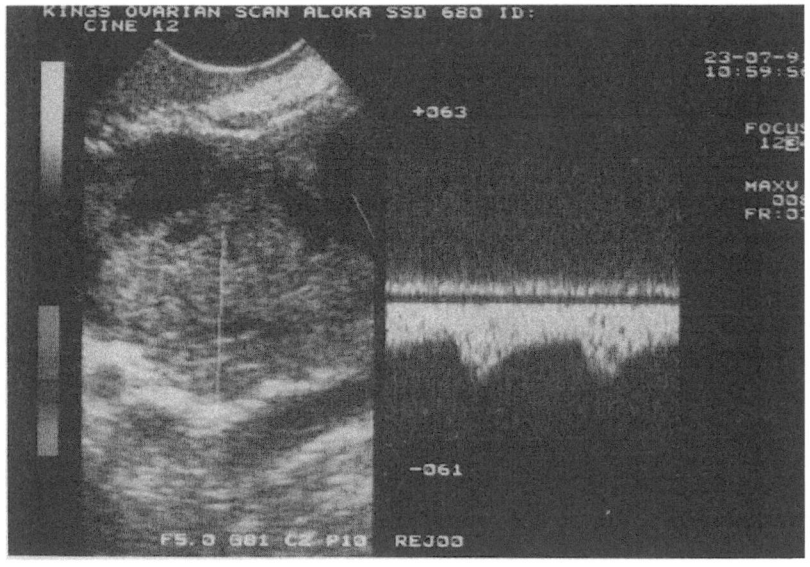

Changes in tissue vascularity are thought to be obligate events in the early stages of ovarian carcinoma, and it has been shown for at least one type of cancer that angiogenesis occurs during the transition from hyperplasia to neoplasia [26]. Transvaginal colour Doppler offers the potential to demonstrate these vascular changes, and thus provide a possible means of discriminating between benign and malignant ovarian lesions (fig 2). Using this technique, the familiar B mode ultrasound image is divided up into many pixels, and the Doppler flow information from each of these pixels is demonstrated on screen in »real-time«. In this way areas of vascularisation can be located as areas of colour. A pulsed Doppler range gate can then be placed over the area of interest to produce flow velocity waveforms that can be analyzed to produce quantitative data. The possible uses and application of transvaginal colour Doppler in gynaecological practice have been described [19]. Preliminary data suggest that it may be possible to detect the vascular changes associated with early ovarian carcinoma, malignant tumours having a characteristic low impedance blood flow pattern [27,28]. Table 1 shows the sensitivity of colour Doppler for the detection of ovarian cancer regardless of stage as well as when it is at stage I. Care must be taken in assessing premenopausal women as neovascularisation is also associated with the developing follicle and corpus luteum [29], whilst after the menopause there are fewer events to confuse the examiner. However despite these relative limitations in our own studies we have observed a reduction in the odds of a women being referred for surgery have been reduced to 1:5 from about 1:15 [30]. It must be remembered that even in a high risk population about 250 women have to be screened to find one carcinoma, so to determine the sensitivity and specificity of colour Doppler as a second stage test for the detection of early ovarian cancer requires a very large database that will only be supplied by multicentre trials.

Conclusions

There are no data currently available to suggest that screening for ovarian cancer will do anything to reduce mortality and morbidity from the disease, only a randomised controlled clinical trial will provide us with this information. Ultrasound provides a screening test for early ovarian cancer which has sufficient sensitivity and specificity for it to used if such a trial is ever carried out. It is obvious that our relative lack of information about the pathogenesis of ovarian cancer makes it difficult to predict what impact screening might have, however given the poor progress that has been made in the treatment of this cancer it seems a reasonable option to try and detect the disease earlier in the hope of altering the outcome for the patient. Transvaginal ultrasonography has the advantage of being able to detect other pelvic malignancies such as endometrial and bladder cancer [31,32], whilst it is a simple matter to take a cervical smear when the patient is positioned for the scan. The natural site for such a service would be alongside existing mammography units so that capital and salary costs could be shared whilst targeting similar groups of women at increased risk. In this way it is possible to imagine a sensible »well women« service for all women around the time of the menopause and beyond.

References

1. Office of Population Censuses and Surveys: Cancer statistics: registrations, England and Wales 1984, HMSO. London, 1988
2. Day T.G., Smith J.P.: Diagnosis and staging of ovarian cancer. Semin. Oncol. 2: 217, 1975
3. Young R.C., Walton L.A., Ellenberg S.S., Homesley H.D., Wilbanks G.D., Decker D.G., Miller A., Park R., Major F. Jr.: Adjuvant therapy in stage I and stage II epithelial ovarian cancers - results of two prospective randomised trials. N. Eng. J. Med. 322: 1021-1027,1990
4. Annual report on cancer statistics
5. Bourne T.H., Reynolds K., Campbell S.: Ovarian Cancer Screening. Eur. J. Cancer 27: 655-659,1991
6. Wilson J.M.G., Jungner G.: In: Principles and Practice of Screening for Disease. Public Health Papers 34, World Health Organisation, Geneva, 1968
7. Cuckle H.S., Wald N.J., In Sharp F., Mason W., Leake R.E., eds.: Ovarian Cancer: Biological and Therapeutic Challenges. Cambridge, Chapman and Hall Medical, 229-239, 1990
8. Daunter B.: Tumor markers in gynecologic oncology. Gynecol. Oncol. 39: 1-15, 1990
9. Jacobs I., Bast R.C.: The CA 125 tumour associated antigen: a review of the literature. Human Reproduction 4: 1-12,1989
10. Zurawski V.R., Orjaseter H., Anderson A., Jellum E.: Elevated serum CA 125 levels prior to the diagnosis of ovarian neoplasia: relevance for early detection of ovarian cancer. Int J. Cancer 42: 677-680, 1988
11. Jacobs I.J., Stabile I., Bridges J., Kemsley P., Reynolds C., Grudzinskas J.G., Oram D.H.: Multimodal approach to screening for ovarian cancer. Lancet, i: 268-271, 1988
12. Zurawski V.R., Sjovall K., Schoenfeld D.A., Broderick S.F., Hall P., Bast R.C., Eklund G., Mattsson B., Connor R.J., Prorok P.C., Knapp R.C., Einhorn N.: Prospective evaluation of CA 125 levels in normal population, phase I: The specificities of single and serial determinations in testing for ovarian cancer. Gynecol. Oncol. 36: 299-305, 1990

13. Campbell S., Goessons L., Goswamy R., Whitehead M.I.: Real time ultrasonography for determination of ovarian morphology and volume - a possible new screening test for ovarian cancer ? Lancet, i: 425-426, 1982
14. Campbell S., Bhan V., Royston P., Whitehead M.I., Collins W.P.:. Transabdominal ultrasound screening for early ovarian cancer. British. Medical Journal, 299: 1363-1367, 1989
15. Campbell S., Bhan V., Royston P., Whitehead M.I., Collins W.P.: Novel screening strategies for early ovarian cancer by transabdominal ultrasonography. Br. J. Obstet. Gynaecol. 97: 304-311, 1990
16. Luxman D., Bergman A., Sagi J., David M.P.: The Postmenopausal Adnexal Mass: Correlation Between Ultrasonic and Pathologic Findings. Obstet. Gynecol. 77: 726-728, 1991
17. Parker W.H., Berek J.S.: Management of selected cystic adnexal masses in postmenopausal women by operative laparoscopy: a pilot study. Am. J. Obstet. Gynecol. 163: 1574-1577, 1990
18. Timor-Trisch I.E., Bar-Yam Y., Elgali S., Rottem S.: The technique of transvaginal sonography with the use of a 6.5 Mhz probe. Am. J. Obstet. Gynecol. 158: 1019-1024, 1988
19. Bourne T.H.: Transvaginal color Doppler in Gynecology. Ultrasound Obstets Gynecol.1: 359-373, 1991
20. Rodriguez M.H., Platt L.D., Medearis A.L., Lacarra M., Lobo R.A.: The use of transvaginal sonography for evaluation of postmenopausal ovarian size and morphology. Am. J. Obstet. Gynecol. 159: 810-814, 1988
21. Van Nagell J.R., Higgins R.V., Donaldson E.S., Gallion H.H., Powell D.E., Pavlik E.J., Woods C.H.: Transvaginal sonography as a screening test for ovarian cancer. A report of the first 1000 cases screened. Cancer 65: 573-577, 1990
22. Bourne T.H., Whitehead M.I., Campbell S., Royston P., Bhan V., Collins W.P.: Ultrasound screening for familial ovarian cancer. Gynecologic Oncology, 43: 92-97, 1991
23. Lynch H.T., Watson P., Bewtra C., Conway T.A., Hippee C.R., Kaur P., Lynch J.F., Ponder B.A.J.: Hereditary ovarian cancer. Cancer 67: 1460-1466, 1991
24. Meire H.B., Farrant P., Guha T.: Distinction of benign from malignant ovarian cysts by ultrasound. Br. J. Obstet. Gynaecol. 85: 893-899, 1978
25. Sassone A.M., Timor-Tritsch I.E., Artner A., Westhoff C., Warren W.B.: Transvaginal sonographic characterisation of ovarian disease: evaluation of a new scoring system to predict malignancy. Obstet. Gynecol. 78: 70-76, 1991
26. Folkman J., Watson J., Ingber D., Hanahan D.: Induction of angiogenesis during the transition from hyperplasia to neoplasia. Nature (London), 339: 58-61, 1989
27. Bourne T.H., Campbell S., Steer C.V., Whitehead M.I., Collins W.P.: Transvaginal colour flow imaging: a possible new screening test for ovarian cancer. British Medical Journal, 229: 1367-1370, 1989
28. Kurjak A., Zalud I.: Early detection of ovarian cancer by transvaginal color Doppler.J. Ultrasound Med. 10: 57, 1991
29. Bourne T.H., Jurkovic D., Waterstone J., Campbell S., Collins W.P.: Intrafollicular blood flow during human ovulation. Ultrasound Obstet. Gynecol. 1: 63-69, 1991

30. Campbell S., Bourne T.H., Reynolds K., Hampson J., Royston P., Whitehead M.I., Collins W.P.: Role of colour Doppler in and ultrasound based screening programme. In Sharp F., Mason W.P., Leake R.E. (Eds) Ovarian Cancer Biological and Therapeutic Challenges, Vol II (Cambridge: Chapman and Hall Medical)
31. Bourne T.H., Campbell S., Royston P., Whitehead M.I., Steer C.V., Collins W.P.: Detection of Endometrial Cancer by Transvaginal Ultrasonography with Color Flow Imaging and Blood Flow Analysis: A Preliminary Report. Gynecologic Oncology 40: 253-259, 1991
32. Granberg S.: Bladder tumors, Ultrasound Obstet. Gynecol. 1: 1991

Acknowledgements

The authors are grateful to both the CRC (Cancer Research Campaign) and the ICRF (Imperial Cancer Research Fund) for financial support, and to Keymed (Southend, UK) and the Aloka Co Ltd (Japan) for the use of their ultrasound equipment.

Dignitätsbeurteilung zystischer Ovarialtumoren mittels Vaginalsonographie

R. Osmers

Ovarialzysten gehören zum physiologischen Bild des prämenopausalen Ovars. Aber sowohl beim Follikel- als auch beim Corpus luteum können Persistenzen vorkommen, die dann den Gynäkologen vor die Problematik der Abgrenzung gegenüber echten Neoplasien stellt. Dies erlangt eine besondere Bedeutung vor dem Hintergrund der Erkennung von klinischen Frühformen des Ovarialkarzinoms. Wenn auch das Risiko hierfür mit zunehmendem Alter steigt, gibt es im Gegensatz zum Korpuskarzinom bisher jedoch keine exakt definierte Risikogruppe. Die gynäkologische Palpation versagt bei kleinen Tumoren, zumal 30% aller Ovarialkarzinome an den Ovarien selbst Tumoren von weniger als 6 cm ausbilden. Nach einer Untersuchung von Barber kann mit einer vaginalen Untersuchung maximal ein Ovarialkarzinom auf 10.000 Untersuchungen erfaßt werden. Zervixzytologien und Douglaspunktionen haben sich als Screeningmethoden ebensowenig wie im Serum bestimmte Tumormarkerspiegel nicht bewährt.

Die sehr ungünstigen 5-Jahres-Überlebensquoten bei Ovarialkarzinomen des Stadiums FIGO III und IV unterstreicht nochmals die Bedeutung der Früherkennung.

Da sich von 366 an der Univ.-Frauenklinik Göttingen ausgewerteten Ovarialkarzinomen 25% unterhalb eines Alters von 40 Jahren befanden, ergibt sich hieraus die Problematik, daß man einerseits funktionelle Tumoren wie Follikel- oder Corpus luteum-Zysten nicht durch eine Operation übertherapieren möchte, andererseits Frühformen des Ovarialkarzinoms und deren Vorstufen adäquat behandeln will. Dies impliziert eine operative Intervention, bei der die Kapsel möglichst intakt bleiben sollte, da eine Ruptur des Ovarialkarzinoms des Stadiums FIGO I nach Baltzer mit einer Verschlechterung der 5-Jahres-Überlebensquote um 30% vergesellschaftet ist. Demgegenüber würde eine Follikelruptur, z.B. durch eine laparoskopische Fensterung, keine wesentliche Gefährdung für die Patientin bedeuten. Hierzu wäre aber eine suffiziente präoperative Dignitätsbeurteilung notwendig.

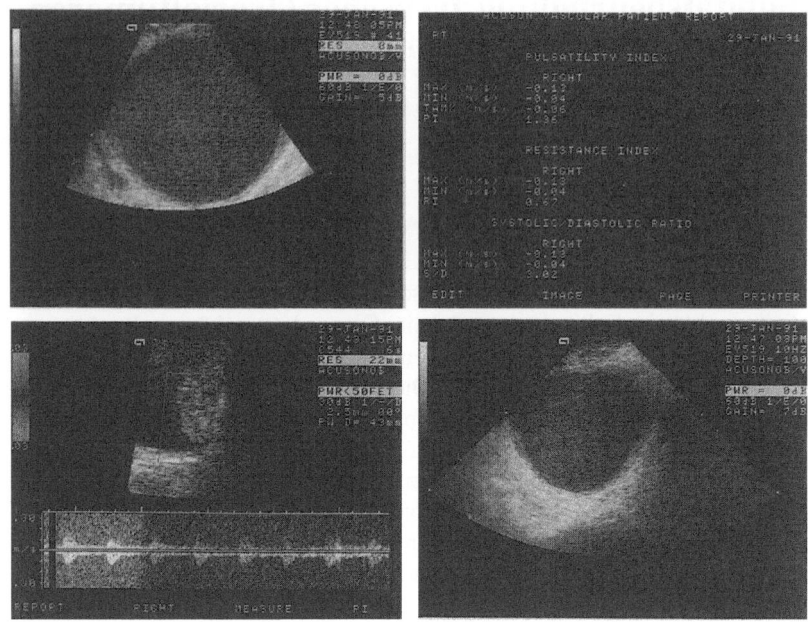

Abb. 1: Einkammerige glattwandige Zyste mit homogenen Binnenechos; Dopplersignal-Ableitung aus einem Gefäß in der Zystenwandung. Histologie: Endometriosezyste. (5,0 MHz, Accuson)

Die Vaginalsonographie bietet sich hierbei als wenig invasives bildgebendes Verfahren und mit einer ausgezeichneten Darstellung pelviner Organe zur Beurteilung der Ovarien an.

Insgesamt haben wir bisher 412 zystische Ovarialtumoren einer Prospektiven sonomorphologischen Beurteilung unterzogen. Wir verwandten hierbei insgesamt fünf sonomorphologische, leicht nachvollziehbare Parameter als Beurteilungskriterien an:

1. Einkammerig-glattwandige Zyste *ohne* Binnenechos
2. Einkammerig-glattwandige Zyste *mit* Binnenechos (Abb. 1)
3. Mehrkammerige Zyste *ohne* Binnenechos in allen Zystenanteilen
4. Mehrkammerige Zyste *mit* Binnenechos in mindestens einem der Zystenanteile
5. Ein- oder mehrkammerige Zysten mit sonographisch solide imponierenden Anteilen (Abb. 2)

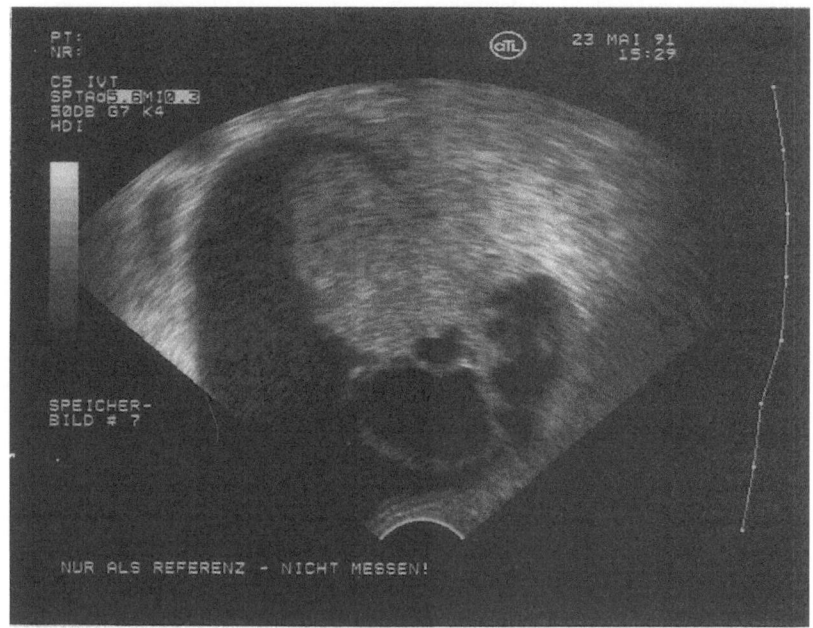

Abb. 2: Mehrkammerige Zyste mit soliden Anteilen. Histologie: muzinöses, papilläres Ovarialkarzinom. (5,0 MHz, ATL, Ultramark 9)

Von den 412 beurteilten Ovarialzysten waren 153 Neoplasien und 259 Retentionszysten, wovon 173 Follikel- und Corpus luteum- und 86 andere Retentionszysten waren (Tabelle 1). Die größte Gruppe bildeten die einkammerigen Zysten ohne Binnenechos mit 130, gefolgt von ein- und mehrkammerigen Zysten mit soliden Anteilen. Derjenige Zystentyp der a priori am ehesten den funktionellen Zysten zugeschrieben wird, fand diese auch in 57% der Fälle, aber mit 21% war jede 5. Zyste dieses sonomorphologischen Typs histologisch einer Neoplasie entsprechend. Der Anteil der Retentionszysten ist mit 22% ausgewiesen. Die sich hieraus ergebende Frage war, inwieweit das Zusatzkriterium Binnenechos innerhalb einer Zyste ein wichtiges sonographisches Kriterium für deren Beurteilung ist. Unsere Untersuchungen ergaben, daß dieses ein Kriterium ist, das keine wesentliche Bedeutung in der Dignitätsabschätzung von Ovarialtumoren hat. Die Blastomfrequenz war mit 21% absolut mit derjenigen der vorangehenden Gruppe identisch. 51% gegenüber 57% funktionellen Zysten in der vorherigen Gruppe weisen ebenfalls keinen wesentlichen Unterschied auf. Das gleiche gilt mit 28% Retentionszysten.

Tabelle 1: Sonomorphologische Beurteilung von zystischen Ovarialtumoren und deren histologisches Korrelat. Inzidenz von echten Neoplasien nach nochmaligem Ultraschall nach 6 Wochen und Befundpersistenz

Sonomorphologie	Follikel- und CL Zysten (n=173)	Sonst. Retentionszysten (n=86)	echte Neoplasien (n=153)
einkammerige Zyste ohne Binnenechos (n=130)	**79%** 57%	22%	**21%** Kontrolle 48%
einkammerige Zyste mit Binnenechos (n=(82)	**79%** 51%	28%	**21%** Kontrolle 43%
mehrkammerige Zyste ohne Binnenechos (n=53)	**62%** 40%	22%	**38%** Kontrolle 63%
mehrkammerige Zyste mit Binnenechos (n=47)	**64%** 30%	34%	**36%** Kontrolle 63%
ein- und mehrkammerige Zyste mit »soliden« Anteilen (n=100)	**28%** 21%	7%	**72%** Kontrolle 91%

Retentionszysten (n=259) Histologie

Bringt das Entscheidungskriterium Mehrkammerigkeit gegenüber Einkammerigkeit einen wesentlichen Gewinn?

Hier läßt sich sagen, daß durch die Diagnose mehrkammeriger zystischer Ovarialtumor die Neoplasiefrequenz von 21 auf 38%, also knapp das Doppelte, gesteigert werden kann. Aber auch in dieser Gruppe beträgt der Anteil der funktionellen Zysten noch immer 40% bei einem wenig veränderten Anteil anderer Retentionszysten mit 22%. Auch hier stellt sich die gleiche Frage, inwieweit Binnenechos in einem oder mehreren Anteilen einer einkammerigen Zyste ein wesentliches Entscheidungskriterium in der Beurteilung hinsichtlich der Dignität von zystischen Ovarialtumoren bildet. Und hier zeichnet sich genauso wie im Vergleich zwischen den beiden einkammerigen Zystengruppen folgender Befund ab:

Beide mehrkammerigen Gruppen wiesen hinsichtlich der Blastomfrequenz mit 36 gegenüber 38% keinen wesentlichen Unterschied auf. Der Anteil der Follikel- und Corpus luteum-Zysten beträgt in dieser Gruppe 30% und der der Retentionszysten 35%. In der letzten Gruppe der ein- und mehrkammerigen Zysten mit solide imponierenden Anteilen sind zwar mit 72% die höchsten Blastomanteile vertreten, aber immerhin sind 21% funktionelle Zysten von 28% Retentionszysten in dieser Gruppe vertreten. Das heißt, daß eigentlich das typische sonomorpholgische Bild der Neoplasien tatsächlich in jedem fünften Fall histologisch einer funktionellen Zyste entspricht.

Das Problem wird noch transparenter, wenn man sich die Sonomorphologie der wichtigsten Ovarialtumoren vor Augen hält:
150 ausgewertete funktionelle Ovarialtumoren wiesen in 67% einkammerigglattwandige Zysten auf, aber in 12% entsprachen sie Zysten mit soliden Anteilen, und in 21% waren sie mehrkammerig. Demgegenüber wiesen zwar alle von uns beurteilten Ovarialkarzinome (n=52) in 92% das sonomorphologische Bild von zystischen Tumoren mit soliden Anteilen auf. Letztendlich waren aber auch 4% einkammerig-glattwandig und 4% mehrkammerig ohne solide Anteile. Dies unterstreicht die Problematik der sonographischen Dignitätsbeurteilung von zystischen Ovarialtumoren. Das seröse Ovarialkystom imponiert zwar sonomorphologisch in 43% ebenfalls als einkammerig-glattwandige Zyste, in 48% kann es auch mehrkammerig sein und weist in 9% die gleichen Kriterien wie 92% aller Ovarialkarzinome und 12% der funktionellen Tumoren auf. Beim muzinösen Ovarialkarzinom sieht man sonographisch in 56% einkammerige Zysten, in 39% mehrkammerige, aber auch ebenfalls in 5% Zysten mit solide imponierenden Anteilen. Endometriosezysten, bei denen häufig ein »typisch« sonomorphologisches Bild einer einkammerigen Zyste mit homogenen feinen Binnenechos nachgesagt wird, weisen diese Kriterien mit und ohne Binnenechos nur in 66% auf. 30% imponieren mehrkammerig, wie auch zahlreiche Neoplasien, und in 4% können selbst strukturelle Ähnlichkeiten mit dem Ovarialkarzinom gesehen werden.

Bildet die sonographisch gemessene Größe von zystischen Ovarialtumoren ein wichtiges Entscheidungskriterium?

Obwohl wir funktionelle Tumoren erst aufgrund einer Kriteriendefinition ab 3 cm Größe in der Postmenopause in unserer Studie erfaßt haben, bildet diese Gruppe mit durchschnittlich 4,5 cm die kleinste Ovarialzystenart. Die Größe variiert jedoch zwischen 3,0 und 11,8 cm. Die mit 29% am häufigsten vertretene Neoplasieart, das seröse Ovarialkystom, weist nahezu identische Größen mit 3,1 - 12,0 cm mittlerem Tumordurchmesser auf. Eine Differenzierung zwischen diesen beiden Befunden wäre aufgrund des etwas größeren durchschnittlichen Tumordurchmessers von 6,3 cm beim serösen Ovarialkystom nicht möglich. Ähnliche Dimensionen weist die sog. Ovarialzyste mit 1,8 - 11,0 cm auf. Etwas größer sind lediglich das muzinöse Ovarialkystom mit 4,7 - 14,4 cm und die Zystadenofibrome mit 3,3 - 16,6 cm Durchmesser. Die größten Tumorvolumina werden bei Durchmessern bis 18,7 cm zwar bei den Ovarialkarzinomen erreicht, aber das kleinste Ovarialkarzinom maß in unserem Untersuchungskollektiv 28 mm. Als Entscheidungskriterium konnten wir herausarbeiten, daß keine funktionellen Zysten oberhalb eines mittleren Tumordurchmessers von 12 cm gefunden werden. Dies hat jedoch letztendlich praktisch keine wesentliche Bedeutung, da nur ein geringer Prozentsatz von 4% größer als 12 cm ist.

Wenn auch resümierend gesagt werden muß, daß mittels Vaginalsononographie keine sichere Differenzierung zwischen funktionellen Ovarialtumoren, Retentionszysten und echten Neoplasien möglich ist, so bietet dennoch die sonomorphologische Beurteilung neben der Klinik ein zusätzliches Entscheidungskriterium zum operativen Vorgehen. Ein abwartendes klinisches Verhalten unter sonographischer Kontrolle innerhalb der nächsten sechs Wochen reduziert die Inzidenz von Follikelzysten auf ein Minimum, wodurch unnötige Operationen weitestgehend vermieden werden können.

Prospektiv bleibt abzuwarten, inwieweit neue sonographische Ansätze wie Farb-Doppler-sonographische Untersuchung in Gefäßen von Ovarialtumoren zu einer weiteren Differenzierung führen können.

Möglichkeiten und Grenzen der Immunszintigraphie in der Diagnostik des Ovarialkarzinoms

R.P. Baum, A. Hertel, J.F. Chatal[*], G. Hör

Definition und technologische Grundlagen

Die Immunszintigraphie wird definiert als eine radio-immunologische Methode zum szintigraphischen Nachweis von zellgebundenen (z.b. tumorassoziierten) Antigenen und wird bei onkologischen Fragestellungen zur Detektion okkulter Tumorrezidive bei ansteigenden Tumormarkern (CA 125 beim Ovarialkarzinom) und im Therapieverlauf (Restaging nach Chemotherapie) eingesetzt [3].

Hierzu werden monoklonale Antikörper (»tausendfache eineiige Zwillinge«) gegen definierte tumorassozierte Antigene mit einem geeigneten Gammastrahler (Radionuklide wie Technetium-99m oder Indium-111) markiert und intravenös appliziert. Die heute klinisch eingesetzten Kitpräparationen müssen hohe Qualitätsansprüche erfüllen (stabile Bindung des Radionuklids an den Antikörper, Erhalt der Immunreaktivität, hohe radiochemische Reinheit, schnelle Markierungstechnik), die von den kommerziell erhältlichen Antikörper-Bestecken erfüllt werden. Ganzkörperuntersuchungen werden mittels regionaler Szintigramme in anteriorer und posteriorer Sicht durchgeführt. Die dreidimensionale Darstellung mittels Emmissions-Computertomographie (SPECT = single photon emission computed tomography) erlaubt eine bessere Lokalisation, Auflösung und Detektion vor allem im Abdomen und kleinen Becken. Die potentiellen Vorteile der Immunszintigraphie sind:

1. Ganzkörperuntersuchung
2. Detektion auch kleiner Tumordeposits (z.B. Peritonealkarzinose)
3. Differenzierung zwischen vitalem Tumorgewebe und Narbe

Abteilung für Nuklearmedizin, Klinikum der Johann Wolfgang Goethe Universität Frankfurt am Main;
[*]Inserm U211, Nantes, Frankreich

Immunszintigraphie beim Ovarialkarzinom mit OC 125

Bedeutsam für die Verbesserung der schlechten Prognose des Ovarialkarzinoms im fortgeschrittenen Stadium (FIGO III, IV), ist das rechtzeitige Erkennen von Rezidiven. Zwar leistet CA 125 hierbei sehr gute Dienste, konventionelle bildgebende Verfahren (CT, NMR, Sonographie) bleiben jedoch im Frühstadium häufig negativ oder inkonklusiv. Daher besitzt CA 125 nach wie vor eine Lead-time (Zeit bis zum Nachweis des vermuteten Rezidivs) von über 3 Monaten. Über den gesicherten Markeranstieg wird die Indikation zur Immunszintigraphie (IS) gestellt, häufig bei fehlender klinischer Symptomatik. Die nuklearmedizinische Rezidivdiagnostik mittels monoklonaler Antikörper (MAK) ist bei dieser (und anderen) Indikationen inzwischen als Routineverfahren anerkannt.

Der murine MAK OC 125 (gerichtet gegen das CA 125 Antigen) wurde 1981 erstmals von Bast et al. beschrieben. Verschiedene immunhistochemische Studien zeigten, daß über 80% der serösen Ovarialkarzinome CA 125 exprimieren. Erhöhte Serum-Spiegel von CA 125 werden bei über 80% der Patienten mit Ovarialkarzinom und bei Rezidiven gefunden. Der MAK OC 125 wurde als Jod-131 und Indium-111 markiertes $F(ab')_2$ Fragment in verschiedenen Studien getestet [2,4]. Chatal et al. berichteten über eine Sensitivität von 72% (chirurgisch und histologisch gesichert) in einer prospektiven Studie [6]. Unsere eigene Gruppe fand eine diagnostische Genauigkeit von 86% bei 33 Patienten [1]. Eine prospektive Multizenter-Studie unter Beteiligung unserer Frankfurter Arbeitsgruppe verglich die Treffsicherheit des Indium-111 markierten OC 125 $F(ab')_2$ mit CT und Ultraschall [7]. Alle Patienten (n=47) waren in Remission nach primärer Operation. Ziel war die Überprüfung der klinischen Wertigkeit der IS in der Diagnose-Strategie beim Ovarialkarzinom im Vergleich mit häufig eingesetzten bildgebenden Verfahren.

Patientencharakteristika

FIGO-Stadium: Ia-II: 23%; Ic,IIc,III: 62%; IV 15%, n= 47 Patienten.
Erhöhter CA-125 Serumspiegel: 44/47 Patienten, 10-5000 U/ml (Mittelwert: 624 U/ml)
CA 125 als einziger Hinweis auf ein Rezidiv: 33 Patienten
CA 125 Erhöhung plus klinische Symptome: 11 Patienten
Normales CA 125, aber klinische Symptome und/oder suspekte CT-Befunde bei 3 Patienten.

Untersuchungstechnik

Die immunszintigraphischen Befunde wurden mittels Histologie (Operation oder Biopsie, 53%) oder durch den klinischen Verlauf (CT, Ultraschall, NMR) bestätigt. Die Patienten erhielten 111 MBq Indium-111 OC 125 F(ab')$_2$, die szintigraphische Untersuchung (planar und SPECT) erfolgte am Injektionstag und 72 Stunden nach Injektion.

Statistik

Unter Anwendung des Bayes' Theorem wurden — ausgehend von zwei unterschiedlichen Prävalenzen (Krankheitswahrscheinlichkeit bei niedrigem CA 125 gleich 0,5, bei deutlich erhöhtem CA 125 gleich 0,7) - die drei bildgebenden Verfahren Röntgen-Computertomographie (CT), Sonographie (US) und Immunszintigraphie (IS) hinsichtlich Sensitivität, Spezifität sowie positivem und negativem Vorhersagewert, einzeln und in Kombination, verglichen.

Ergebnisse

Tabelle 1 gibt die Ergebnisse für alle Verfahren wieder. Die Werte, die sich bezüglich der Sensitivität und der Spezifität ergaben sind aus Tabelle 2 ersichtlich. Die sich aus diesen Ergebnissen errechneten positiven und negativen Vorhersagewerte (PPV, NPV) für eine niedrige Prävalenz (0,5) sind in Tabelle 3 aufgeführt.

Tabelle 1: Ergebnisse von IS, CT, US (Anzahl der Befunde beim Gesamtkollektiv)

	RP	FN	FP	RN	Gesamt
IS	33	2	4	8	47
CT	11	9	2	5	27
US	12	16	3	5	36

IS=Immunszintigraphie, CT=Computertomographie, US=Ultraschall
RP= richtig positiv, FN= falsch negativ, FP=falsch positiv, RN= richtig negativ

Tabelle 2: Sensitivität und Spezifität von IS, US, CT

	US	CT	IS
Sensitivität	43	55	94
Spezifität	62	71	67

Tabelle 3: PPV und NPV bei niedriger Prävalenz (50%)

	US	CT	US+CT	IS	US+IS	CT+IS	US+CT+IS
PPV	53	65	66	74	76	84	86
NPV	52	61	63	92	92	94	95

Stellenwert der Immunszintigraphie in der Nachsorge des Ovarialkarzinoms

Als bedeutendes Ergebnis dieser prospektiven Untersuchung kann festgehalten werden, daß der *negative Vorhersagewert der IS sehr hoch* ist (92%) und durch Ultraschall und CT nicht mehr gesteigert werden kann. Klinisch praktisch bedeutet dies, daß *bei fraglichem Ovarialkarzinom-Rezidiv* (z.B. schwankender Verlauf der CA 125 Serumwerte, d.h. Krankheitsprävalenz 0,5) die *Immunszintigraphie als alleiniges Verfahren* ausreicht, um ein *Rezidiv auszuschließen*. Hingegen reichen Ultraschall und CT nicht aus, um ein Rezidiv sicher auszuschließen (negativer prädiktiver Wert 63% von US+CT).

Der *positive Vorhersagewert* der Immunszintigraphie liegt deutlich höher (74%) als für Ultraschall und CT zusammengenommen (66%). Für einen ausreichenden positiven Vorhersagewert (0,84) müssen CT und IS positiv sein. Für die Praxis bedeutet dies, daß bei *vermutetem Ovarialkarzinomrezidiv* und *positiver Immunszintigraphie* eine *Röntgen-Computertomographie ergänzend* durchgeführt werden sollte, um das Rezidiv zu bestätigen. Die Immunszintigraphie war von allen drei Verfahren das akkurateste (Sensitivität und Spezifität kombiniert).

Abb. 1: Okkulte, linksseitige subdiaphragmale Metastase eines Ovarialkarzinomrezidivs vom Borderlinetyp (Erstoperation 1987. Jetzt ausstrahlende Schmerzen in die linke Schulter beim Husten!). Immunszintigramm von Thorax/Abdomen in posteriorer Sicht, Technetium-99m B 43.13 Anti-CA 125 MAK 24 Stunden nach Applikation.

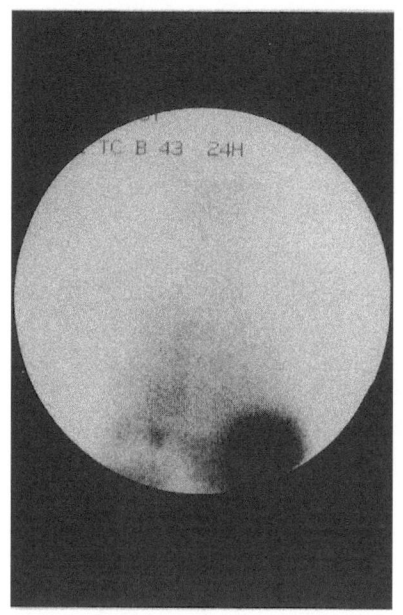

Bezüglich der therapeutischen Strategie war die IS als einziges Verfahren in 18 Fällen wegweisend, davon konnte bei 9 Patienten 8 mal eine vollständige Tumorresektion durchgeführt werden. Drei Patienten konnte eine Operation wegen des ausgedehnten Befalls im Immunszintigramm erspart werden.

Neben dem In-111 markierten OC 125 MAK ist mittlerweile auch ein Technetium-99m markierter MAK gegen CA 125 in klinischer Prüfung (B43.13), der durch die wesentlich kürzere Halbwertzeit des Technetiums (6 Stunden, Indium zum Vergleich 2,8 Tage) bei deutlich reduzierter Strahlenexposition höhere Aktivitäten und damit eine bessere Auflösung ermöglicht. Durch die geringere unspezifische Speicherung in der Leber wird auch eine Evaluierung von Lebermetastasen möglich (Abb. 1 und 2). Erste Erfahrungen unserer Arbeitsgruppe zeigten vergleichbar gute Ergebnisse wie beim OC 125 in der Rezidivdiagnostik [5].

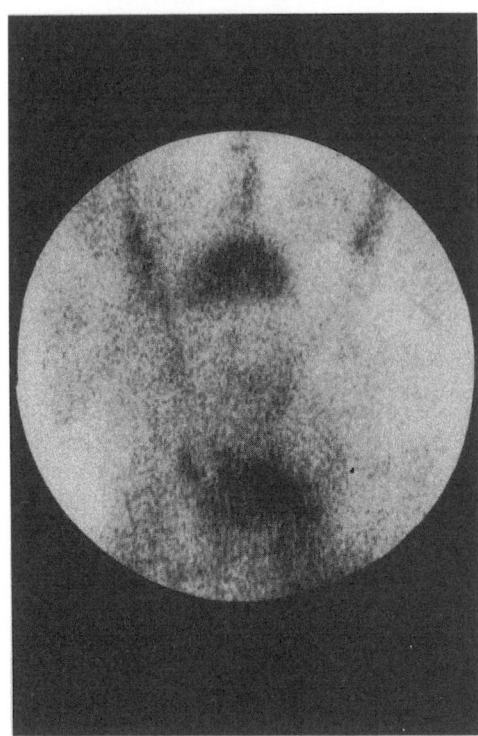

Abb. 2: Peritonealkarzinose mit Infiltration der Abdominalwand bei deutlich erhöhtem CA 125 im Serum (132 U/ml). Sonographisch / computertomographisch wurde lediglich ein Aszites als möglicher Hinweis auf eine peritoneale Aussaat beschrieben. Immunszintigramm des Abdomens (anterior) mit Technetium-99m B 43.13 24 Stunden nach Applikation.

Grenzen und Probleme der Immunszintigraphie

Einschränkungen bezüglich einer beliebigen Wiederholbarkeit der IS betreffen vor allem die Bildung von humanen Anti-Maus Antikörpern (HAMA), die durch HAMA-MAK Komplexbildungen und rascher Speicherung im RES der Leber eine erfolgreiche Antigenbindung am Tumor verhindern. Potentielle allergische Komplikationen können durch konsequentes Messen der HAMA vor und 6 Wochen nach jeder Applikation vermieden werden [9]. Bei deutlich erhöhten und lange Zeit persistierenden HAMA-Werten sollte eine erneute Szintigraphie nicht mehr durchgeführt werden. Die Entwicklung chimärer (teils murines, d.h. von der Maus abstammendes Protein der Antigenbindungsstelle, teils humanes IgG) oder humaner Antikörper (nur noch humames Protein) wird in Zukunft die HAMA-Problematik lösen helfen.

Die Bildung von HAMA nach Szintigraphie mit MAK gegen CA 125 kann zu massiven Störungen von in vitro Assays mit falsch positiven oder massiv falsch positiven CA 125 Werten führen [10]. Verantwortlich für diesen Störeffekt sind anti-idiotypische HAMA (gegen die Antigenbindungsstelle gerichtet), die in den Assays fälschlicherweise als CA 125 erkannt werden [8,12]. Die Verwendung differenter CA-125-Assays oder Entfernen von HAMA aus dem Serum kann diesen Effekt umgehen. Gleichzeitig beobachteten wir und die Bonner Arbeitsgruppe bei Patienten mit diesem Phänomen eine ungewöhnlich lange Überlebenszeit trotz schlechter Prognose (FIGO III, IV oder Rezidive) [11,13]. Möglicherweise bewirken die durch die IS induzierten HAMA über weitere Antikörper oder T-Lymphozyten einen suppressiven Effekt an der Tumorzelle.

Schlußfolgerungen

Die Immunszintigraphie sollte unbedingt in die Rezidivdiagnostik integriert werden, bei Rezidivverdacht und negativem Ultraschall (indiziert, da schnell und einfach durchführbar) sollte zunächst die Immunszintigraphie erfolgen, um bei suspekten Befunden eine gezielte CT zu veranlassen. So würde durch eine sinnvolle Kombination aller drei bildgebenden Verfahren eine Optimierung der Rezidiverkennung im frühest möglichen Stadium mit anschließender potentiell kurativer Sekundärintervention (Operation, Second line Chemotherapie, Immuntherapie) möglich.

Literatur

1. Baum R.P., Lorenz M., Senekowitsch R. et al.: Clinical experience in cancer diagnosis with radiolabeled monoclonal antibodies in 200 patients and inital attempts at radioimmunotherapy. In: Srivastava, S.C. (Ed.) Radiolabeled monoclonal antibodies for imaging and therapy. Plenum Publishing Cooperation, 1988
2. Baum, R.P., Hertel A., Hör G.: Immunszintigraphische Diagnostik in der Nachsorge gynäkologischer Karzinome. Gynäkologe 22: 33-38, 1989
3. Baum, R.P., Hör G.: Immunszintigraphie gynäkologischer Tumoren. In: Käser O., Friedberg V., Ober K.G., Thomsen K., Zander J. (Hrsg.): Handbuch Gynäkologie und Geburtshilfe, Bd III/2 Spezielle Gynäkologie 2. Friedberg V., Thomson K. (Hrsg.), 2. Auflage, Thieme, Stuttgart-New York 24.48-24.55, 1988

4. Baum, R.P., Chatal J.F., Fumoleau P. et al.: Results of an European Multicenter Study on immunoscintigraphy with In-111-DTPA OC 125 F(ab')2 in gynecological tumors. In: Schmidt H.A.E., Buraggi G.L. (Eds.): Trends and Possibilities in Nuclear Medicine. Schattauer, Stuttgart-New York: 679-682, 1989
5. Baum R.P., Hertel A., Baew-Christow T., Noujaim A., Hör G.: A novel Tc-99m labeled monoclonal antibody against CA 125 (B43.13) for radioimmunodetection of ovarian cancer - Initial results. Eur. J. Nucl. Med. 18: 535, 1991
6. Chatal, J.F. (Ed.): Monoclonal Antibodies in Immunoscintigraphy. CRC Press, Boca Raton, 1989
7. Dutin J.P., Peltier P., Chatal J.F.: Bayesian Analysis of the Utility of In-111 OC 125 Immunoscintigraphy (IS) in Diagnosing Ovarian Cancer. J. Nucl. Med. 32: 941, 1991
8. Hertel A, Baum R.P., Auerbach B., Herrmann A., Hör G.: A simple procedure to detect anti-idiotypic human anti-mouse antibodies (HAMA) after immunoscintigraphy. FK Schattauer, Stuttgart, New York 159-161, 1990
9. Hertel A., Baum R.P., Auerbach B., Herrmann A., Hör G.: Klinische Relevanz humaner Anti-Maus-Antikörper (HAMA) in der Immunszintigraphie. Nucl. Med. 29: 221-227, 1990
10. Hertel A., Baum R.P., Auerbach B., Herrmann A., Hör G.: Effects of Human Anti-Mouse Antibodies (HAMA) on Tumor Marker Assays. In: R. Klapdor (ed) Recent Results in Tumor Diagnosis and Therapy, Zuckschwerdt Verlag München, Bern Wien San Francisco: 461-463, 1990
11. Hertel A., Baum R.P., Baew-Christow T., Schulte L., Hör G.: Anti-idiotypic HAMA Triggered by OC 125 Radioimmunoscintigraphy: Beneficial To The Patient? Proceedings Hamburger Tumormarkersymposium, Dezember 1991 (in press)
12 Muto M.G., Lepisto E.M., van den Abbeele A.D., Knapp R.C., Kassis A.I.: Influence of human antimurine antibody on CA 125 levels in patients with ovarian cancer undergoing radioimmunotherapy or immunoscintigraphy with murine monoclonal antibody OC 125. Am. J. Obstet. Gynecol. 161: 1206-1212, 1989
13. Wagner U., Reinsberg J., Oehr P., Briele B., Schmidt S., Werner A., Krebs D., Biersack H.J.: Clinical course of patients with ovarian carcinomas after induction of anti-idiotypic antibodies against a tumor-associated antigen. Tumor Diagnostik & Therapie 11: 1-4, 1990

Aussagekraft von sonographischen und computertomographischen Staging Untersuchungen bei Ovarialkarzinomen

A. Vering, J. Peters[*], H.G. Bender

Abstract

Bildgebende Verfahren zur präop. Einschätzung der Tumorausdehnung sind eine wichtige Planungsgrundlage zur Therapie bei abdominalen Tumoren, wobei die Patientenbelastungen bzw. Kosten bei der Computertomographie (CT) höher sind, als bei der Ultraschalluntersuchung (US). Inwieweit sich dies durch exaktere Ergebnisse rechtfertigt, sollte in dieser Studie geprüft werden.

Patienten
Es wurden 45 Patientinnen mit gynäkologischen Malignomen untersucht, davon 25 mit Ovarialkarzinomen. Die Ergebnisse wurden soweit möglich mit den intraoperativen bzw. histologischen Befunden verglichen.

Ergebnisse
Eine fast vollständige Deckungsgleichheit der CT und US Befunde fand sich hinsichtlich der Parameter Lebermetastasen, Aszitesbildung, Aufstau der Nieren und Tumorausbreitung im kleinen Becken. Retroperitoneale Lymphknoten wurden allenfalls durch CT erkannt. Die Vorhersage von Tumoranteilen außerhalb des kleinen Beckens ließen sich mit der CT nur geringfügig exakter nachweisen. Bei Adipositas verliert der US seine Aussagekraft zum Teil.

Schlußfolgerung
In unserer Studie zeigte sich eine erstaunlich hohe Korrelation der beiden bildgebenden Verfahren in der globalen Einschätzung fortgeschrittener Ovarialkarzinome.

Zentrum der Frauenheilkunde und Geburtshilfe
[*]Zentrum der Radiologie

Einleitung

Zur präoperativen Planung bei Patientinnen mit Verdacht auf Ovarialkarzinom werden in der Regel sowohl Ultraschall (US), als auch Computertomographie (CT) durchgeführt. Dabei wird der CT im klinischen Alltag eine wesentlich höhere Wertigkeit zugebilligt, oftmals kann die konkrete Operationsplanung erst nach Vorliegen der CT beginnen. Leider vergehen auch in großen Kliniken oft mehrere Tage, bevor eine CT durchgeführt werden kann. Es erschien uns jedoch erstaunlich, wieviele der relevanten Befunde auch schon in der meist einige Tage früher durchführbaren US Untersuchung erkennbar und bewertbar waren, sodaß wir uns zu einem systematischen Vergleich der Aussagekraft beider Verfahren entschlossen.

Material und Methoden

Es wurden im Rahmen dieser Studie die Befunde von 25 Ovarialkarzinomen des Stadiums III (n=19) bzw. IV (n=6) verglichen, die durch US und CT erhoben wurden. Von diesen Patientinnen konnten 17 laparotomiert werden.

Die Ultraschalluntersuchungen wurden durch 2 erfahrene Untersucher in einem weitgehend standardisierten Untersuchungsgang mit dem Acuson 128 durchgeführt. Die Tumordarstellung wurde zunächst im kleinen Becken begonnen, wobei sowohl abdominal (3,5 MHz) als auch vaginalsonographisch (5 MHz) mit einer Sektorsonde untersucht wurde. Dabei wurde die Struktur und Ausdehnung des Tumors genau beschrieben, sowie die Beziehung zur Beckenwand sowie den Nachbarorganen Blase und Rektum dargestellt. Anschließend wurde abdominalsonographisch der gesamte Bauchraum nach eventuell vorliegenden Tumoranteilen und / oder Aszitesbildung untersucht und zum Schluß beide Nieren sowie die Leber. Eine systematische sonographische Darstellung eventueller retroperitonealer Lymphknotenmetastasen wurde bei den hier vorgestellten Patientinnen nicht vorgenommen.

Besonderer Wert wurde auf eine exakte Dokumentation der erhobenen Befunde mit Bildern bzw. Dias gelegt, um die Befunde auch demonstrieren zu können.

Die CT Untersuchungen wurden durch erfahrene Radiologen im Rahmen der Tumorbesprechung demonstriert und befundet.

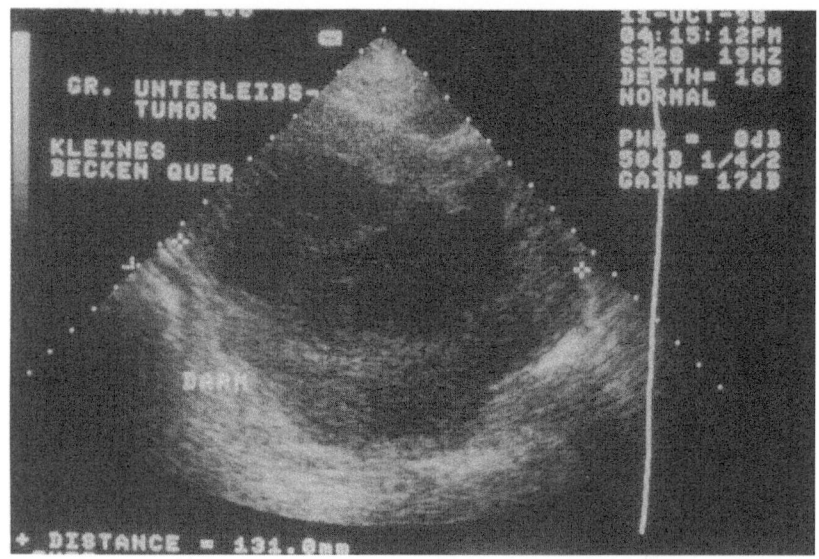

Abb. 1: Vergleich eines sonographischen und computertomographischen Querschnittes durch das kleine Becken bei einem Ovarialkarzinom Stadim IV.

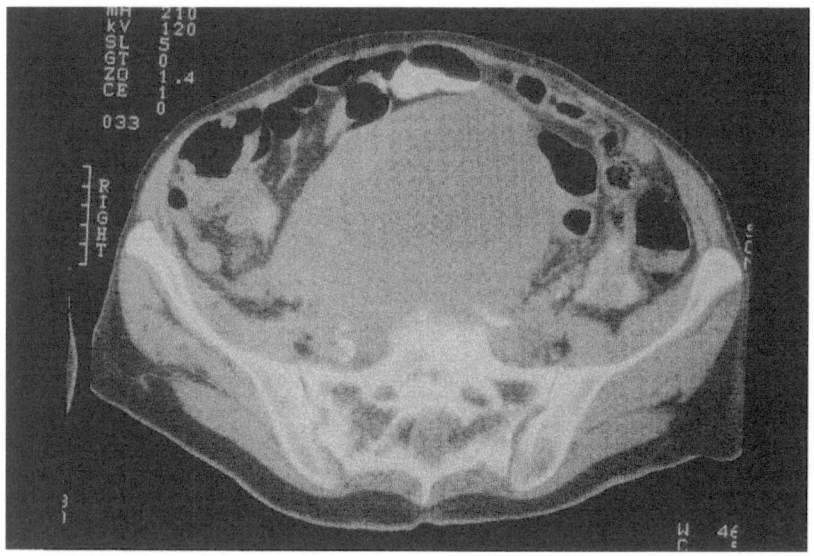

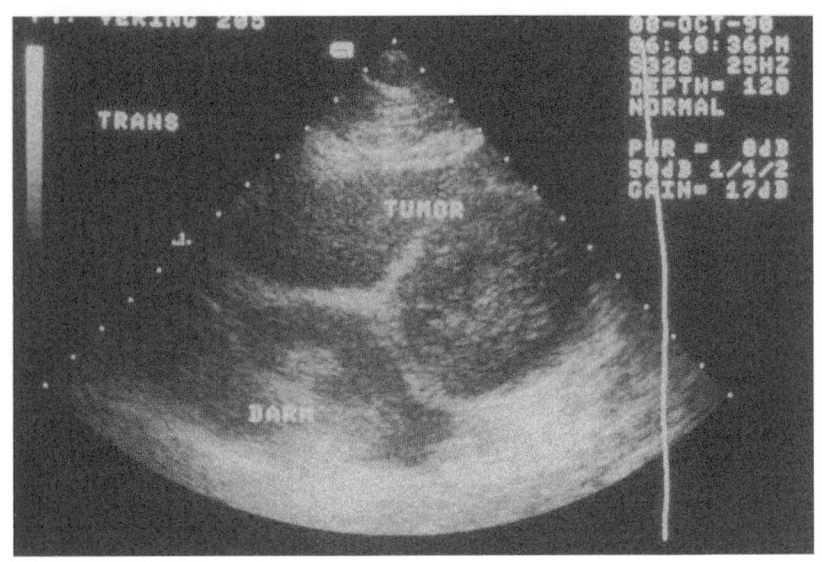

Abb. 2: Ileuszustand bei Ovarialkarzinom Stadium III

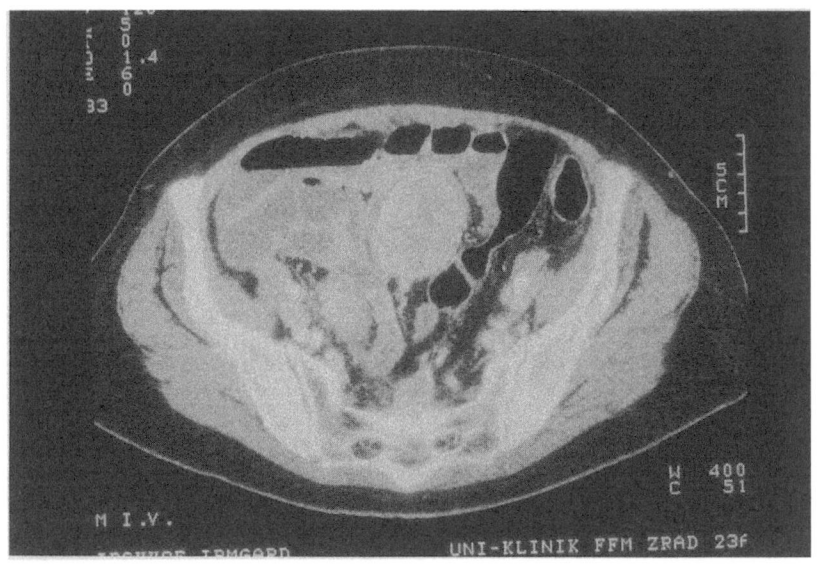

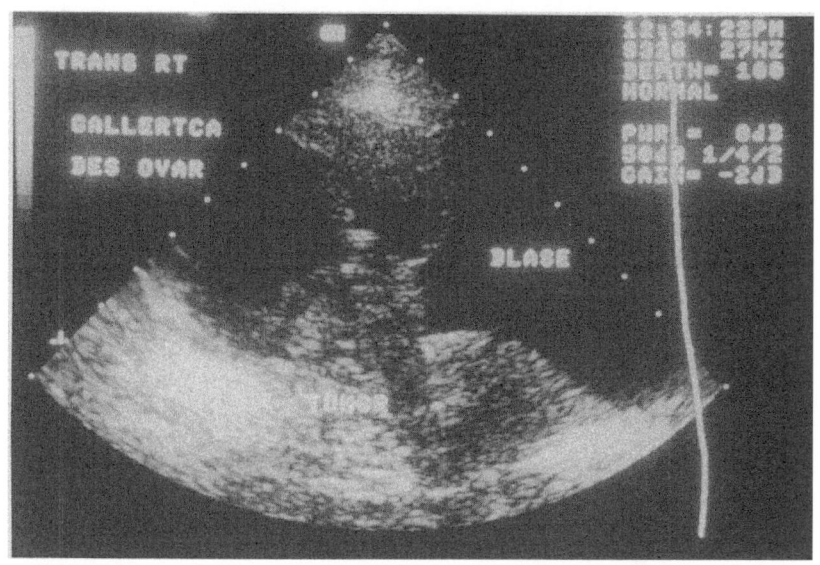

Abb. 3: Sonographische und computertomographische Darstellung der teils soliden, teils cystischen Struktur eines Rezidivs eines Gallertkarzinoms des Ovars.

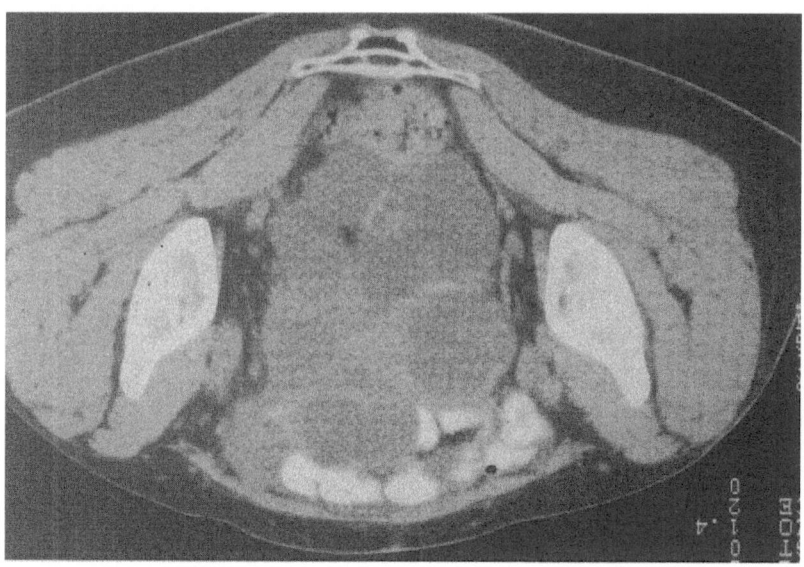

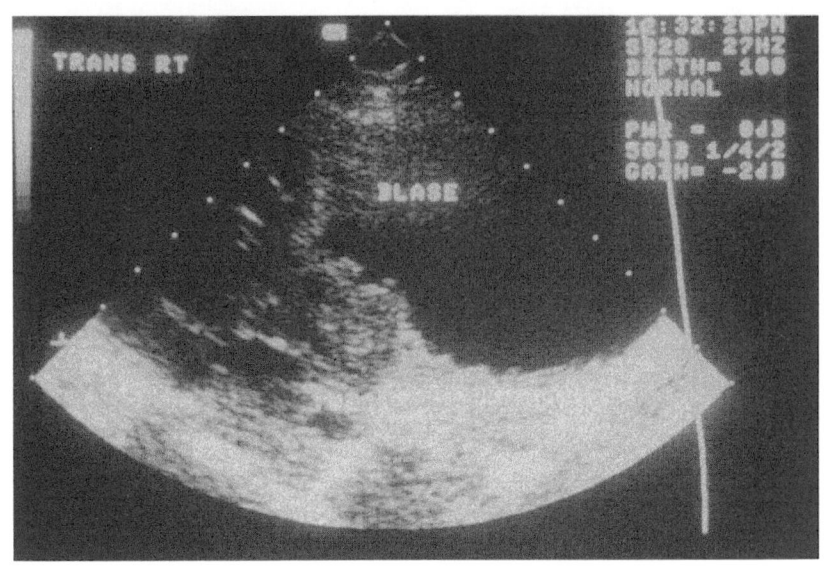

Abb. 4: Demonstration der Blaseninfiltration im Ultraschall und der Computertomographie.

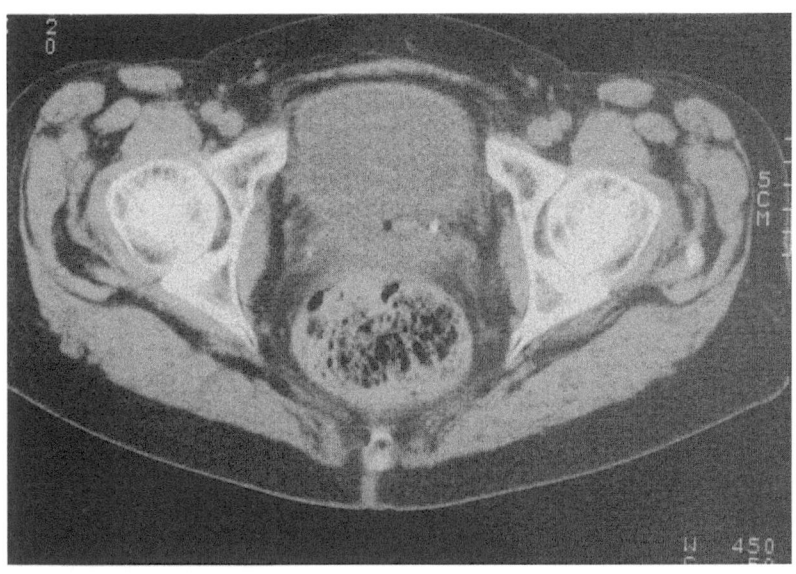

Tabelle 1

korrekte prätherapeutische Beurteilung	US(n)	CT(n)	Klinisch oder histologisch verifiziert
Aszites	19	19	19
Aufstau des Nierenbeckens	6	6	6
Lebermetastasen	4	5	5
Tumorausbreitung im kleinen Becken	11	12	17
Tumorausbreitung im Abdomen	4	6	10
Retroperitoneale LK	0	2	6

Ergebnisse

Wie in Tabelle 1 aufgeführt, konnte bei 19 von 25 Patientinnen mit Ovarialkarzinomen des Stadiums III und IV durch beide Verfahren eine klinisch verifizierte Aszitesbildung nachgewiesen werden. Auch die Diagnostik der ableitenden Harnwege konnte mit beiden Verfahren sehr exakt durchgeführt werden. In einem Falle einer adipösen Patientin wurde sonographisch eine Lebermetastasierung übersehen, die in der CT gesehen wurde und durch den Verlauf bewiesen wurde. Beide Verfahren können die Tumorausbreitung im kleinen Becken mit guter Genauigkeit vorrausagen, wobei sich im Zuge der Laparotomie, in 3 (CT) bzw. 4 (US) Fällen eine Überbewertung der Tumorausdehnung fand und in jeweils 2 Fällen eine Unterbewertung. Allerdings ist die Operabilität der Ovarialkarzinome nur bedingt aus der Tumorausdehnung zu erschließen.

Wesentlich ungenauere Ergebnisse werden mit beiden Methoden bezüglich der Tumorausdehnung im gesamten Bauchraum gefunden, wobei die CT hierbei Vorteile bietet. Retroperitoneale Lymphknotenmetastasen konnten in dieser Studie nur durch die CT gefunden werden, allerdings war hierbei die Sensitivität auch nur gering.

Diskussion

Die Ultraschalluntersuchung kann bei fortgeschrittenen Ovarialkarzinomen bezüglich der Parameter Aszitesbildung, Aufstau des Nierenbeckens und Lebermetastasen eine Genauigkeit erbringen die der der Computertomographie vergleichbar ist. Eine nahezu gleichwertige Genauigkeit beider Verfahren fand sich in unserem kleinen Kollektiv bzgl. des Parameters Tumorausbreitung im kleinen Becken. Allerdings weisen beide Verfahren hier doch eine weniger optimale Übereinstimmung mit den Befunden auf, die anläßlich der Laparotomie erhoben werden können. Noch nicht ganz befriedigend sind die Ergebnisse beider Methoden bezüglich der Parameter »Tumorausbreitung im Bauchraum« und »Retroperitoneale Lymphknotenmetastasierung«, wobei sich allerdings Vorteile für die CT ergeben. Insgesamt verliert die US Untersuchung bei Adipositas der Patientinnen in stärkerem Maße ihre Aussagekraft als die CT.

Aus unserer Untersuchung ergeben sich somit folgende Schlußfolgerungen. Die Ultraschalluntersuchung ist meist wesentlich schneller verfügbar und kann durchaus für die operative Planung bei Ovarialkarzinomen benutzt werden. Die Computertomographie wird dennoch die Standardmethode bleiben, da sie in Einzelfällen doch aussagekräftiger und der Untersuchungsgang besser standardisierbar ist. Die Ergebnisse der CT sind außerdem im Standbild besser demonstrierbar.

MIX
Papier aus verantwortungsvollen Quellen
Paper from responsible sources
FSC® C105338

If you have any concerns about our products,
you can contact us on
ProductSafety@springernature.com

In case Publisher is established outside the EU,
the EU authorized representative is:
**Springer Nature Customer Service Center GmbH
Europaplatz 3, 69115 Heidelberg, Germany**

Printed by Libri Plureos GmbH
in Hamburg, Germany